ANA
AMERICAN NURSES ASSOCIATION

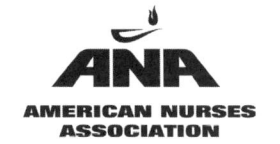

Scope AND **Standards** OF PRACTICE | # Home Health Nursing

2ND EDITION

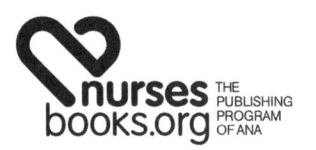

nursesbooks.org
THE PUBLISHING PROGRAM OF ANA

American Nurses Association
Silver Spring, Maryland
2014

American Nurses Association
8515 Georgia Avenue, Suite 400
Silver Spring, MD 20910-3492
1-800-274-4ANA
http://www.Nursingworld.org

Published by Nursesbooks.org
The Publishing Program of ANA
http://www.Nursesbooks.org/

The American Nurses Association (ANA) is a national professional association. This publication, *Home Health Nursing: Scope and Standards of Practice, Second Edition*, reflects the thinking of the practice specialty of home health nursing on various issues and should be reviewed in conjunction with state board of nursing policies and practices. State law, rules, and regulations govern the practice of nursing, while *Home Health Nursing: Scope and Standards of Practice, Second Edition,* guides home health nurses in the application of their professional skills and responsibilities.

The American Nurses Association is the only full-service professional organization representing the interests of the nation's 3.1 million registered nurses through its constituent/state nurses associations and its organizational affiliates. The ANA advances the nursing profession by fostering high standards of nursing practice, promoting the rights of nurses in the workplace, projecting a positive and realistic view of nursing, and by lobbying the Congress and regulatory agencies on healthcare issues affecting nurses and the public.

Copyright © 2014 American Nurses Association. All rights reserved. Reproduction or transmission in any form is not permitted without written permission of the American Nurses Association (ANA). This publication may not be translated without written permission of ANA. For inquiries, or to report unauthorized use, email copyright@ana.org.

ISBN-13: 978-1-55810-559-1   SAN: 851-3481   1.5K   07/2014

First printing: July 2014

Contents

Contributors	vii
Introduction	ix
Scope of Practice of Home Health Nursing	1
Evolution of Home Health Nursing	1
Home Health Nursing's Scope of Practice	4
Definition of Home Health Nursing	5
Distinguishing Characteristics of Home Health Nursing	6
The Nursing Process in Home Health Nursing	7
Assessment	7
Diagnosis	8
Outcomes Identification	8
Planning	9
Implementation	9
Evaluation	10
Educational Preparation of Home Health Nurses	10
Certification in Home Health Nursing	11
Practice Roles and Responsibilities	11
Home Health Nurse	11
Graduate-Level Prepared Home Health Nurse	13
Advanced Practice Registered Nurse	13
Clinical Nurse Specialist	13
Nurse Practitioner	14
Clinical Roles	15
Care or Case Manager	15
Patient Educator	16
Patient Advocate	17

CONTENTS

Administrative Roles	18
Administrator	18
Supervisor or Clinical Manager	19
Quality and Performance Improvement Nurse	20
Clinical Educator	20
Informatics Liaison Nurse	22
Trends, Issues, and Opportunities in Home Health Nursing	23
Practice Environments	23
Ethics in Home Health Nursing	27
Respect for the Individual	27
Commitment to the Patient	27
Advocacy for the Patient	28
Responsibility and Accountability for Practice	28
Duties to Self and Others	29
Contributions to Healthcare Environments	29
Advancement of the Nursing Profession	30
Collaboration to Meet Health Needs	30
Promotion of the Nursing Profession	31
Research in Home Health Nursing	31
Informatics in Home Health Nursing	35
Finances and Reimbursement	39
Summary of the Scope of Home Health Nursing Practice	41

Standards of Home Health Nursing Practice — 43
Significance of the Standards — 43

Standards of Practice for Home Health Nursing — 44
Standard 1. Assessment — 44
Standard 2. Diagnosis — 46
Standard 3. Outcomes Identification — 47
Standard 4. Planning — 49
Standard 5. Implementation — 51
   Standard 5A. Coordination of Care — 53
   Standard 5B. Health Teaching and Health Promotion — 54
   Standard 5C. Consultation — 56
   Standard 5D. Prescriptive Authority and Treatment — 57
Standard 6. Evaluation — 58

Standards of Professional Performance for Home Health Nursing   60
    Standard 7. Ethics   60
    Standard 8. Education   62
    Standard 9. Evidence-Based Practice and Research   64
    Standard 10. Quality of Practice   65
    Standard 11. Communication   67
    Standard 12. Leadership   68
    Standard 13. Collaboration   70
    Standard 14. Professional Practice Evaluation   72
    Standard 15. Resource Utilization   73
    Standard 16. Environmental Health   75

Glossary   77

References   79

Appendix A. *Home Health Nursing: Scope and Standards of Practice* (2007)   87

Index   155

Contributors

A special thank you to the volunteer members of the ANA workgroup for their time and excellent work in revising the 2014 edition of *Home Health Nursing: Scope and Standards of Practice*.

Workgroup

Marilyn D. Harris, MSN, RN, NEA-BC, FAAN, Chairperson

Lisa Gorski, MS, HHCNS-BC, CRNI, FAAN

Patricia Hanks, MS, RN, COS-C

Patricia M. Hunt, MS, RN

Karen S. Martin, MSN, RN, FAAN

Mary Narayan, MSN, RN, HHCNS-BC, CTN, COS-EC

Maria Radwanski, MSN, RN, CRRN

The work group that created this 2014 revision of *Home Health Nursing: Scope and Standards of Practice* gratefully acknowledges the work of the previous task forces of 2007, 1999, 1992, and 1986 that initiated the original documents on home health nursing.

Reviewers

Deborah Center, MSN, RN, CNS

Joann K. Erb, PhD, RN

Tina M. Marrelli, MA, RN, MSN, FAAN

Imelda A. Nwoga, MSc, RN, MSN, PhD

ANA Staff

Carol J. Bickford, PhD, RN-BC, CPHIMS – Content editor
Maureen E. Cones, Esq. – Legal counsel
Yvonne Daley Humes, MSA – Project coordinator
Eric Wurzbacher, BA – Project editor

About the American Nurses Association

The American Nurses Association (ANA) is the only full-service professional organization representing the interests of the nation's 3.1 million registered nurses through its constituent/state nurses associations and its organizational affiliates. The ANA advances the nursing profession by fostering high standards of nursing practice, promoting the rights of nurses in the workplace, projecting a positive and realistic view of nursing, and by lobbying the Congress and regulatory agencies on healthcare issues affecting nurses and the public.

About Nursesbooks.org, The Publishing Program of ANA

Nursesbooks.org publishes books on ANA core issues and programs, including ethics, leadership, quality, specialty practice, advanced practice, and the profession's enduring legacy. Best known for the foundational documents of the profession on nursing ethics, scope and standards of practice, and social policy, Nursesbooks.org is the publisher for the professional, career-oriented nurse, reaching and serving nurse educators, administrators, managers, and researchers as well as staff nurses in the course of their professional development.

Introduction

Home Health Nursing: Scope and Standards of Practice, Second Edition, describes the professional practice of all home health registered nurses. This scope statement and these updated standards and competencies of home health nursing practice are meant to define, guide, and direct home health professional nursing practice.

The American Nurses Association (ANA) has been active in the development of nursing scope and standards of practice since the late 1960s. ANA published the first standards, *Standards of Nursing Practice*, for the nursing profession in 1973. These standards were generic in nature and focused on the basic nursing process—a critical thinking model applicable to all registered nurses and nursing—composed of assessment, diagnosis, outcomes identification, planning, implementation, and evaluation. Various revisions have ensued, the most recent being *Nursing: Scope and Standards of Practice, Second Edition* (ANA, 2010a), which is to be used in conjunction with *Nursing's Social Policy Statement: The Essence of the Profession* (ANA, 2010b) and *Code of Ethics for Nurses with Interpretive Statements* (ANA, 2001). These three resources provide a complete and definitive description of nursing practice and nursing's accountability to the public in the United States.

Specialty nursing organizations have affirmed the 2010 ANA scope and standards publication by using the template language of the standards and accompanying competencies when developing scope of practice statements and standards of practice for registered nurses in specialty practice. ANA published the first of these, *Standards of Home Health Nursing Practice*, in 1986; a revision followed in 1992. The 1999 revision, *Scope and Standards of Home Health Nursing Practice*, included a scope of practice statement to describe the specialty practice as well as its revised standards of practice.

As part of its regular process of development, review, and maintenance of scope and standards of specialty nursing practice, ANA convened a volunteer workgroup of home health nursing professionals in 2013 to review and revise the 2007 specialty scope and standards to better reflect contemporary home health nursing practice and provide a framework for future practice. Registered nurses (RNs) and advanced practice registered nurses (APRNs) in different home health settings and in various roles responded to ANA's call for volunteers. The workgroup:

- Assessed research reports, publications, and evidence-based practice.

- Distributed and sought input on the updated draft scope and standards from nurses who attended the Home Healthcare Nurses Association (HHNA) meetings at the National Association for Home Care and Hospice (NAHC) annual meetings in October 2013.

- Shared information and requested input from nurses through a guest editorial in *Home Healthcare Nurse* (Harris, 2013).

- Requested input on the document from ANA's Constituent Member Associations (CMAs), specialty nursing organizations, home health organizations, and other stakeholders.

- Posted the draft document on ANA's web site for public review and comment by interested nurses and others.

The workgroup considered all public comments and suggestions in preparing the final document for submission to the ANA review process. Reviews by ANA's Committee on Nursing Practice Standards and Board of Directors culminated in the final edits, acknowledgment of the scope of practice, approval of the standards of practice, and publication of *Home Health Nursing: Scope and Standards of Practice, Second Edition*.

Scope of Practice of Home Health Nursing

Evolution of Home Health Nursing

Community-based care, including home health nursing, has been provided for centuries. Florence Nightingale, William Rathbone, and their colleagues, formalized home health practice in England during the 1800s, selecting the titles of district nurses (home health) and health visitors (public health), which are still in use in the United Kingdom. Both *Notes on Nursing* (Nightingale, 1859) and *A Guide to District Nurses and Home Visiting* (Craven, 1889) shaped American nurses' goals to formalize home visiting programs in the United States.

Nurse home visiting was conducted by both lay and trained nurses beginning in the early 19th century in many cities and towns in the United States. After mid-century, Roman Catholic and Protestant sisters and deaconesses across the country were joined by dedicated women providing home nursing services through local churches or settlement houses. These services continued even as secular trained nurses were increasingly employed by new voluntary organizations growing out of the charity organizing movement, beginning in the mid-1880s in New York City, Buffalo, Philadelphia, and Boston (Dieckmann, 2012). Known as visiting nurse associations or services, these local agencies were generally led by boards of prominent, wealthy women concerned about their community's health and social services.

Early nurse leaders, including Lillian Wald, Lavinia Dock, Margaret Sanger, and Mary Breckinridge, refined and publicized diverse models of health promotion and disease prevention. In the late 1800s Visiting Nurse Associations (VNAs) and the nursing divisions of governmental health agencies, such as city and county health departments, provided the majority of services. Community health nurses, as generalists, gave nursing care to the sick, as well as health promotion services to individuals, families, and communities. Public health principles and practice, and components of family and community care, were integrated into home-based nursing services.

Several key events drove the steady but slow growth of home care in the early 1900s. In 1909 the Metropolitan Life Insurance Company created an innovative program that paid for nurses to care for its policyholders in the home, prompting other life insurance companies to provide this critical service as well. During World War II, as physicians made fewer home visits and focused instead on providing care in offices and hospitals, the home care movement grew, with nurses providing most of the health and illness care services in the home. In 1946, Montefiore Hospital in New York City developed a post-hospital acute care program and initiated convalescent home care (Buhler-Wilkerson, 2003, 2012).

In 1952, the American Nurses Association (ANA) and the National League for Nursing (NLN) became the primary national nursing organizations, following the merger and restructuring of other organizations. The NLN became the primary membership organization for nurses practicing in the community for the next 30 years.

At mid-20th century, improvements in care and treatment of acute illness had revealed the need to address the burden of chronic illness on Americans through disease-specific prevention, screening, medical management, and rehabilitation (Commission on Chronic Illness, 1956–1959). Both visiting nurse and official agencies expanded home visiting to include rehabilitation, with new emphasis on a multidisciplinary team that included physical, occupational, and speech therapies; social services; and nursing assistants (later called home health aides).

The 1965 Social Security Amendments that introduced Medicare (Title XVIII) included a home health benefit, increased the reach and visibility of home health care, and led to significant growth in this field. Because of the new reimbursement benefits, physicians and hospitals began to discharge patients earlier. In 1976, after 10 years of Medicare services, home health remained at just 1% of total annual reimbursements. The potential for creative expansion of home health services was constrained by congressional amendments and administrative controls that decreased Medicare's focus on post-hospital services.

When the Centers for Medicare & Medicaid Services (CMS) phased in the diagnosis-related groups (DRGs) hospital reimbursement model during the early 1980s, shorter hospital stays became the norm and the need for home care services expanded. Home health nurses were thus faced with providing highly complex clinical care for patients in the patients' homes. New treatments and technology enabled more patients to be treated at home, resulting in increased referrals to existing agencies and the establishment of many new agencies, some affiliated with hospitals and some independent, proprietary enterprises. Home health nursing practice emphasized acute care in the home, and some agencies began to offer services 24 hours a day, 7 days a week.

With the growth in home health care, CMS attempted to rein in costs through changes in the reimbursement method by establishing the prospective payment system (PPS) and through additional regulations and oversight of home health agency practices. These measures prompted organizational mergers, new reimbursement and quality specialists, and new models for delivering care. The Visiting Nurse Associations of America (VNAA) and the National Association for Home Care and Hospice (NAHC) were formed to help home health agencies address these challenges. These two organizations became the primary specialty advocacy organizations for home health agencies, and continue to provide strong national leadership.

Responding to the expansion of nursing services provided in the home and the need to formalize this specialty practice, ANA published the first version of its practice standards, *Standards of Home Health Nursing Practice*, in 1986. *Scope of Practice for Home Health Nursing* was published in 1992, followed by the combined and expanded *Scope and Standards of Home Health Nursing Practice* in 1999 and another revision in 2008.

Looking forward to 2020, home health nurses will be caring for a more diverse patient population with:

- More families and communities in need of health promotion and disease prevention services

- More infants, children, and adults surviving with deficits from severe illnesses and/or injuries

- More patients who will request palliative and hospice nursing services

- More older adults with multiple chronic diseases, illnesses, and more complex needs

- Increased numbers of people who have joined the ranks of the "very old"

- More patients of differing cultures and languages

- More patients, families, and communities wanting greater choices and care personalized to their needs

Reimbursement for home health care services and models of care will continue to shift and change as the provisions of the 2010 Patient Protection and

Affordable Care Act (ACA) and the vision of the 2010 Institute of Medicine (IOM) report, *The Future of Nursing*, are implemented. Home health nurses will expand their services related to patient engagement, patient-centered care, best evidence-based practices, and care coordination, including across healthcare settings. In addition, home health nurses will assume an even more integral part in making health care less costly, more efficient, and more effective through enhanced use of advanced practice registered nurses, transition-of-care models, and new ways of engaging patients with motivational interviewing and coaching techniques.

The impact of the changing world—globalization, emerging infections, pandemics, natural and manmade disasters, communication and technological advances, economic changes—will have implications for home health nurses and the care they provide. Transitioning patients along the care continuum to the setting that most efficiently, effectively, comfortably, and cost-effectively meets their needs (which is frequently the patient's home) will be a paramount concern.

The home and community are increasing in importance as the recommended point of care delivery. With the speed of technologic advances in medical procedures and efforts directed at satisfying a well-informed public, the home health industry needs to push forward to exceed expectations for care delivery in the community. This involves efforts to define the future goals of home health care. Home health nurses are strategically poised to lead in accountable care, transitioning care from acute settings, and collaborating with other care providers, the patient, and the patient's family. These nurses develop individually suited home- and community-based care plans and instruct, guide, coach, and support the patient and family in achieving the best possible outcomes while remaining in the communities they value.

Home Health Nursing's Scope of Practice

According to the Bureau of Labor Statistics (2010), about 140,000 nurses work in home health nursing, a practice setting predicted to outpace the growth of other settings in the coming decades. These professional nurses should incorporate the updated content of this home health nursing document into practice. The goal of home health nursing is to improve the health, well-being, and quality of life of all home health patients, their families, and other caregivers, and to help people to remain in their homes. This can best be accomplished through the significant and visible contributions of registered nurses using standards and evidence-based practice.

Definition of Home Health Nursing

Home health nursing is a specialty area of nursing practice that promotes optimal health and well-being for patients, their families, and caregivers within their homes and communities. Home health nurses use a holistic approach aimed at empowering patients, families, and caregivers to achieve their highest levels of physical, functional, spiritual, and psychosocial health. Home health nurses provide nursing services to patients of all ages and cultures and at all stages of health and illness, including end of life.

This new home health nursing definition reflects the workgroup's thoughtful discussion and consensus decision-making about the importance of describing home health nursing today and for the future. Public comment during the development and review process affirmed the new definition.

Home health nursing is nursing practice applied to patients of all ages in the patients' residences, which may include private homes, assisted living, or personal care facilities. Although there are multiple terms to identify the recipient of home health nursing services—*patient, client, customer, healthcare consumer*—this document uses the term *patient*. Patients and their families and other caregivers are the focus of home health nursing practice.

The goal of care is to maintain or improve the quality of life for patients, their families, and other caregivers, or to support patients in their transition to end of life. These goals are accomplished by building relationships and engaging the patient, family, and other caregivers through the provision of direct patient care and the promotion of independence, accountability, and self-care. Additionally, the home health nurse, through interprofessional collaboration, initiates, coordinates, manages, and evaluates the resources needed to enhance and promote the patient's optimal level of well-being, capabilities, and independence. Nursing activities necessary to achieve these goals use evidence-based practices and may include preventive, maintenance, restorative, and rehabilitative interventions to prevent potential problems, manage existing health problems, improve clinical outcomes, and prevent hospital and other inpatient admissions and readmissions.

Although the term *home care* is used by many national associations and publications, the professional title of home health nurse is defined and recognized by the nursing profession, other healthcare professionals, and the public. The workgroup members involved in this scope and standards revision considered the terms *home care nurse* and *home health care nurse* and concluded that the title and tradition of *home health nurse* should be continued.

Distinguishing Characteristics of Home Health Nursing

Home health nursing is a specialized area of nursing practice that focuses on individuals in need of care in their homes, their families, and their caregivers. Home health nurses provide care to patients across the lifespan, from the prenatal through the postdeath periods. Home health nursing practice embraces primary, secondary, and tertiary prevention; assistance to families with coordination of community resources and health insurance benefits; and delivery of healthcare services in a patient's home, including nonconventional residences. Home health nursing stresses the holistic management of personal health practices for the treatment of diseases or disability.

Home health nursing reflects more than a change in location or acute care services delivered in the home. Home health requires a change in the definition and structures of care to reflect a broad array of coordinated services, benefits, and caregivers available to patients experiencing complex problems. Home health nurses who care for these patients practice independently and require highly developed skills in assessment and care coordination. Although home health nurses practice in collaboration with other healthcare professionals, they frequently are the only professionals in the home actually providing care to the patient. As such, they must be expert in assessment, clinical decision-making, and clinical practice. These skills form the foundation for definition of outcomes, planning, nursing care interventions, evaluation, communication with other interprofessional healthcare team members, and referral to other healthcare settings when appropriate.

Home health patients may require nursing care resources 24 hours a day, 7 days a week. The frequency and duration of these services is dependent upon the home care delivery model and holistic needs of the unit comprised of the patient, family, and other caregivers. Home health nurses may provide services ranging from intermittent visits to full-time extended daily care. Home health nurses also provide important assistance and guidance for patients and families in decision-making about how best to meet identified needs.

Another distinguishing characteristic of home health nursing is its emphasis on patient and caregiver teaching. The goal of home health nursing is to enable patients and their caregivers achieve independent self-management of the patient's illness, disease, or disability. Thus, the home health nurse provides education and counseling so the patient and caregiver have the knowledge, skills, and abilities to achieve this independence. Home health nurses assess learning needs, learning styles, and health literacy. They teach about health promotion, disease prevention and management, medications, safety, and resource access. Home health nurses provide counseling and coaching to help patients and their caregivers adapt and cope with the lifestyle changes necessitated by chronic illnesses and disabilities. They use the principles of adult learning and evaluate learning using teach-back and return-demonstration techniques.

Home health nursing differs from other nursing specialties in the degree of responsibility nurses assume in managing the financial cost of care. Home health nurses work directly with public and private payors and with consumer-directed payment programs. Home health nurses must have advanced knowledge of reimbursement systems to help patients obtain the care they need while containing the cost of care.

The Nursing Process in Home Health Nursing

Home health nurses use the nursing process, the essential methodology by which patient goals are identified and achieved. The nursing process, comprised of assessment, diagnosis, outcomes identification, planning, implementation, and evaluation, is used throughout clinical care, administration, education, research, quality improvement, and other home health practice areas. (The nursing process is also the basis for the Standards of Practice for Home Health Nursing, which are set out in the next section.)

Assessment

Home health nurses assess the physical, psychosocial, and environmental factors that affect a patient's health. In addition, they perform in-depth functional assessments and medication assessment.

Physical assessment includes interviewing patients and their caregivers about the patient's health history and diagnoses, and includes performing a complete physical assessment of all the patient's body systems and capabilities, along with a review of nutritional needs.

Psychosocial assessment includes assessing the patient's cognitive, developmental, behavioral, and coping status and includes screening for anxiety, depression, and abuse or neglect. This assessment also addresses social support systems and spiritual needs. Furthermore, a psychosocial assessment discovers the patient's language preference, health literacy, learning style, and cultural needs and preferences. Special attention is paid to the multiple impacts the patient's illness and disease have on the family, the caregiver, and the patient's/family's finances.

Environmental assessment focuses on risks within the home and community to the patient's and home health clinician's personal health and safety. A home environmental assessment includes attention to obstacles within the home that may increase the risk for falls (e.g., throw rugs, clutter), presence of needed safety features (e.g., grab bars in the bathroom, rubber bathmats), presence of smoke alarms, and safety practices that are required for home treatments, such as oxygen safety. Sanitation issues that may affect the risk of infection are also assessed. Some examples of clinician safety issues to be addressed include presence of latex in the home for those with allergies, pet issues, and presence of firearms in the home (National Institute for Healthcare Safety and Health [NIHSH], 2010).

Home health nurses perform comprehensive *medication assessments*, which include reconciling medications in the home to the prescriber's list and the patient's diagnoses; monitoring the medications for effectiveness, side effects or adverse effects, and interactions; assessing the ability of the patient and the caregiver(s) to safely and consistently administer the medications; and identifying any barriers or issues related to medication adherence.

Home health nurses also perform comprehensive *functional assessments* to determine the patient's risk for falls and ability to safely perform activities of daily living (ADLs) and independent activities of daily living (IADLs), including the ability of the patient and caregiver(s) to safely manage all medical/assistive devices and equipment.

Diagnosis

Home health nurses derive their diagnoses and identify problems from the assessment data. Diagnoses can be focused on the physical, psychosocial, cultural, spiritual, environmental, economic, and interpersonal aspects of care. Home health nurses, in collaboration with the patient, the family, other caregivers, and interprofessional team members, identify actual problems as well as situations that might become problems if unattended.

Outcomes Identification

The home health nurse partners with the patient, family, and other caregivers to identify specific, measureable, attainable, relevant, and time-defined (SMART) goals for the patient based on the patient's identified problems and diagnoses (Doran, 1981). In home health, these goals are the expected patient outcomes: the results of the care by the home health nurse and the interprofessional team. Ideally, the ultimate goal of the plan of care is to return the patient to the highest possible level of self-care within the community. This involves preparing the patient and caregivers to be independent in self-management of disease and other identified problems. However, sometimes the goal is comfortable end-of-life care.

Planning

Home health nurses develop a plan of care in collaboration with the patient, family and other caregivers, and other healthcare providers. This plan is based upon the comprehensive assessment; identified diagnoses, problems, or issues; and expected outcomes or goals. Drawing upon evidence-based strategies and best practices to develop the plan of care, the home health nurse adapts the plan to incorporate and meet the unique needs, preferences, and goals of the patient and caregiver(s).

When the need for other services and supplies is identified, the home health nurse collaborates with the interprofessional home health team to further develop the most effective and economical plan. When the goal of discharging the patient back to the community and self-care cannot be achieved, ongoing home health care may be provided and revisions to the plan of care are made. In addition, home health nurses are engaged in education, administration, and research activities, which also require planning.

Implementation

Home health nurses implement the plan and provide skilled nursing interventions to patients, as well as patients' families and caregivers, including direct care, teaching, counseling, coaching, care management, and resource coordination. In collaboration with the patient, family, and other caregivers, home health nurses determine the most appropriate care strategies, which may include complementary therapies and culturally sensitive approaches, to meet identified patient needs and support achievement of expected outcomes.

Teaching and coaching of the patient, family, and caregiver(s) are integral to the implementation component of the nursing process for home health nurses. Teaching supports the achievement of patient outcomes and the movement of the patient and the family toward engagement and independence. As patient educators, home health nurses use a variety of media and strategies to develop and reinforce enhanced self-care skills. Home health nurses provide information about community health resources to patients, patients' families, and other caregivers. Through this information exchange and advocacy, including effective teach-back and return-demonstration techniques, home health nurses engage patients, families, and other caregivers in planning for and seeking additional services as their needs dictate.

The home health nurse assesses the implementation of the care plan and care provided by the licensed practical nurse/licensed vocational nurse (LPN/LVN) and home health aide. Although the LPN/LVN and home health aide may be team members in the home health setting, the registered nurse provides ongoing assessment and supervision to help ensure positive outcomes. When the patient receives services from multiple practitioners, including nonprofessionals, home health nurses often assume the role of case or care manager and coordinate efforts of all the involved stakeholders, including the patient's primary care provider and other caregivers, to optimize patient outcomes.

Evaluation

The evaluation of patient outcomes provides critical data from which to determine the effectiveness of the plan. Evaluation is an ongoing and dynamic process. The home health nurse evaluates progress toward expected outcomes and thus determines the effectiveness of the plan of care. As the patient's status changes and new data are collected, modifications of the plan of care may be required.

Educational Preparation of Home Health Nurses

Home health nursing, because of its level of independence in practice, requires registered nurses to have a strong foundation of knowledge and expertise. Completion of the baccalaureate nursing degree is the appropriate and preferred educational preparation for home health nurses because of the curricular emphasis on public/community health principles and practice, case management, patient teaching, and leadership. Neal-Boyan (2001), with a consortium of Home Healthcare Nurses Association members (Harris, 2001), developed a core curriculum addressing program management, concepts and models, disease management, and trends, issues, and research, followed by a later publication in 2011 describing "paradigm" home care clinical case studies.

Every nurse entering the specialty must complete an extensive orientation program to master the numerous competencies of the home health nurse. Structured preceptor programs, support from colleagues, clinical experiences, and lifelong learning through academic and continuing education programs promote this professional growth and enhance the ability of both new and experienced home health nurses to assume evolving home health nursing roles and meet the expanding demands of this specialty practice. Associate-degree and diploma nurses who work in home health nursing are strongly encouraged to seek additional education to meet qualifications at the baccalaureate level.

Certification in Home Health Nursing

Because home health nursing is characterized by specialized knowledge, skills, and competencies that are needed to care for patients in the unique setting of patients' homes, achievement of home health nursing or other specialty certification demonstrates such competence to employers and patients. However, at the time of publication, the previously offered American Nurses Credentialing Center (ANCC) home health nurse and home health clinical nurse specialist certifications are no longer available. Certified home health nurses may continue to retain this certification by meeting the continuing education recertification process requisites. Exploratory discussions about an alternative home health nursing certification mechanism are under way. However, home health nurses can also affirm their competence, knowledge, and skills through other nursing certifications, such as in oncology, infusion, wound care, diabetes, pediatrics, hospice and palliative care, psychiatric-mental health, and gerontological nursing.

Practice Roles and Responsibilities

The diverse roles, responsibilities, and functional areas detailed in this section identify some of the clinical and leadership positions in home health nursing. These roles may overlap and complement each other depending on the size of the home health organization, number of staff, and services provided.

Home Health Nurse

Home health nurses provide nursing care in accordance with *Nursing: Scope and Standards of Practice, Second Edition* (ANA, 2010a), as well as the more detailed and specific home health nursing standards. Competent home health nursing practice requires flexibility, creativity, and innovative approaches to problem-solving in the context of individual and environmental differences and resource availability.

Effective home health nursing practice includes identification of and attention to environmental, economic, familial, and cultural characteristics. In addition, a fundamental understanding of psychosocial and safety issues affecting patients, families, and other caregivers is critical for the effective delivery of home health nursing. Because patients residing in their homes may receive healthcare services from an array of providers, home health nurses often assume the role of case or care manager and coordinator. Therefore, the preferred minimum qualifications for a registered nurse practicing in home health nursing are:

- A baccalaureate degree in nursing

- A desire and ability to motivate patients, families, and caregivers in health promotion and disease management by applying change theory, learning principles, and teaching skills

- An ability to apply critical thinking to physical, psychosocial, environmental, cultural, family, and safety issues

- An ability to utilize clinical decision-making in applying the nursing process to care of patients in their homes

- An ability to practice as an effective member of an interprofessional team

- An ability to apply case/care management, communication, and collaboration principles and skills to provide care in the home health setting

- An ability to work within different organizations' payment models while advocating for optimal outcomes for patients

Home health nursing is an autonomous practice requiring additional knowledge and skills beyond those acquired in basic baccalaureate nursing educational programs. The requisite knowledge base and skills for home health nursing can be further developed through individualized formal orientation programs, structured preceptor programs, guided clinical experience based on the specific learning needs of the nurse, and graduate education. Each home health nurse must build and maintain the professional knowledge, skills, and abilities that support evidence-based practice, clinical decision-making, and effective teaching that empower the patient to attain self-management and achieve the best outcomes possible. The employing agency also has an obligation to establish an environment conducive to such professional development.

Graduate-Level Prepared Home Health Nurse

A home health nurse may have completed master's or doctoral level education to accrue advanced knowledge, skills, abilities, and judgment associated within one or more nursing or other specialties. Home health nurses function at an advanced level, as designated by elements of their position in such practice areas as administration, education, research, informatics, and quality improvement. For instance, those who have completed a course of study for a master's of business administration (MBA), master's of health administration (MHA), or other graduate management degree are well prepared for policy, executive, and organizational leadership positions.

Advanced Practice Registered Nurse

Advanced practice registered nurses (APRNs) hold a master's or doctoral degree in nursing, are expert clinicians and consultants, and advance nursing and home health practice by contributing to home healthcare research and by educating and mentoring undergraduate and graduate clinicians. As the Institute of Medicine *Future of Nursing* report (IOM, 2010) indicates, APRNs are needed to augment healthcare services, including in home health. The need and opportunities for APRNs in home health care—especially clinical nurse specialists and nurse practitioners—are immense (IOM, 2010; McClelland, McCoy, & Burson, 2013; Auer & Nirenberg, 2008). APRNs specializing in the needs of home health patients and special populations (e.g., pediatrics, geriatrics) and disease management specialties (e.g., cardiac, diabetes, psychiatric-mental health, and wounds) can improve and enhance the outcomes of home health patients.

Advances have been made in the collaborative role of APRNs working with home health registered nurses and prescribing clinicians. Evolving practice permits the clinical nurse specialist or nurse practitioner who is not directly practicing in home health to collaborate with the certifying physician in accordance with state law and perform the initial home health certification by documenting the required face-to-face encounter with the patient. With the need to develop new care delivery services as the healthcare system evolves, APRNs will find autonomous, creative, and innovative ways to meet the continuity-of-care, transitional, and palliative care needs of patients seeking home-based care.

Clinical Nurse Specialist

The clinical nurse specialist (CNS) is an expert in evidence-based nursing practice, treating and managing the health concerns of patients, families, groups, communities, and populations. In home health care, CNS practice is targeted toward achieving quality, cost-effective outcomes in three spheres of influence (National Association of Clinical Nurse Specialists [NACNS], 2010):

Patient care. CNSs provide comprehensive assessments, expert care, care planning, and care management, including pharmacologic and nonpharmacologic treatments, for home health patients, families, and groups with specific or complex needs. They provide care using evidence-based clinical interventions.

Nurses and nursing practice. CNSs meet the educational needs of nurses and interprofessional colleagues through formal and informal teaching methods. They promote evidence-based practice and consult with staff and administration to improve clinical outcomes.

Organization or system. CNSs act as change agents, initiating innovative programs and quality improvement strategies to enhance the programs and processes of home health agencies and the healthcare systems of which they are a part. They develop and implement evidence-based, best-practice models, and pioneer programs to achieve the safest, most efficient, effective, and economical care for the organization's patient population.

Nurse Practitioner

Nurse practitioners (NPs) are prepared to diagnose and treat patients with undifferentiated symptoms, as well as those with established diagnoses. Initial, ongoing, and comprehensive care includes:

- Taking comprehensive histories, and providing physical examinations and other health assessment and screening activities

- Diagnosing, treating, and managing patients with acute and chronic illnesses and diseases

- Prescribing pharmacologic and nonpharmacologic therapies, including durable medical equipment

- Making appropriate referrals for patients and families

Opportunities for nurse practitioners in home health practice are expected to increase substantially because of healthcare reform and other initiatives. Their ability to practice to the full scope of their education, abilities, and licensure will become even more important and valued in the home care setting.

Clinical Roles

CARE OR CASE MANAGER

The care or case manager role involves not only the delivery of direct care to the patient, but also coordination of and with the care provided by other disciplines. When a patient is admitted to service, the nurse care manager uses the nursing process to assess the patient's unique situation, and develops a plan of care (POC) in consultation with the patient, family, caregivers, team members, and the physician. The home health nurse implements the POC, continually evaluating the patient's progress toward goal achievement, and making plan-of-care adjustments to enable the patient to achieve the highest possible level of health, well-being, and function. Specific activities in this process include:

- Performing a comprehensive holistic assessment that integrates input from the patient, family, and other caregivers, as well as other pertinent sources of information about the patient

- Developing the POC while considering the patient's unique strengths and limitations, and the impact of cultural and religious beliefs on the patient's cognitive, physical, psychosocial, and emotional condition

- Prioritizing care based on mutual goal-setting and outcome identification by the patient and the nurse

- Providing direct care to patients, including ongoing assessment of condition, education of the patient and the family, evaluation of effectiveness of care, and revision of POC to achieve the patient's optimal health potential

- Completing accurate documentation to advocate for needed clinical and other services

- Delegating care to licensed practical nurses and home health aides (HHAs) utilizing the principles of delegation, and providing ongoing instruction and supervision as needed

- Determining the appropriate utilization of services and acknowledging financial parameters when developing and implementing a POC that promotes optimal patient outcomes

- Evaluating the effectiveness of care and the patient's progress toward goals and revising the POC as needed to help the patient achieve optimal potential and positive outcomes, which may include dying with dignity

- Collaborating with the interprofessional team and community resources and maintaining communication related to the patient's response to the POC
- Collaborating with healthcare providers by communicating changes in condition and progress toward goal attainment

PATIENT EDUCATOR

Home health nurses educate patients, families, other caregivers, and the community. Home health nurses provide health coaching and instruction to patients, families, and other caregivers in self-care skills to improve and manage patients' acute and chronic conditions. In this role, nurses share information, demonstrate techniques, and evaluate performance of procedures by patients, families, and other caregivers. It is critically important that the home health nurse assess and address potential barriers to learning effective self-care management. Such barriers may include depression, limited health literacy, cognitive impairment, sensory deficits, functional impairments, and low self-efficacy (Suter, Gorski, Hennessy, & Suter, 2012).

The home health nurse must partner with the patient and family in identifying realistic and achievable goals, thus increasing not only knowledge but also motivation and confidence in the ability to change. Teaching strategies should include use of simple language (avoiding complex words), motivational interviewing and coaching techniques, and use of strategies such as teach-back and return demonstrations to evaluate both teaching by the nurse and learning by the patient (White, Garbez, Carroll, Brinker, & Howie-Esquivel, 2013). The use of action plans that provide patients with guidance in identifying symptoms and actions to take is an effective strategy (Registered Nurse Association of Ontario, 2010). Nurses must assess and respect cultural and religious values, health beliefs, and practices within the process of patient education on healthy lifestyle, health promotion, and disease prevention for patients, families, and other caregivers.

Nurses may also conduct community education programs and provide information about available home health services and reimbursement systems for care. Home health nurses educate physicians and other health professionals about opportunities to work collaboratively in the home setting. The goals for collaboration include helping the patient achieve optimal function, maintain independence, and remain at home in the community.

PATIENT ADVOCATE

One of the primary responsibilities of home health nurses is patient advocacy, which must be incorporated into all steps of the nursing process, not merely during implementation of the plan of care and associated therapies. Patient advocacy includes assisting patients in navigating the healthcare delivery system, supporting them in making healthcare decisions, and helping them access community resources to support independence. Informing, supporting, and affirming the decision-making of patients and their families and other caregivers are important adjuncts to achieving patient care objectives and patient goals.

The home health nurse is often the health professional who interacts directly with patients, patients' families, and other caregivers. As a result of this interaction, nurses frequently become aware of problems or circumstances that interfere (or may interfere) with a patient's recovery, safety, or well-being. Home health nurses treat the individual in a holistic manner and recognize when additional clarification or support is needed or additional resources are required. Nurses may also identify factors that interfere with a patient's recovery, safety, or adherence to the treatment plan. As advocates, home health nurses serve as a liaison between the patient, the family (as providers of care), other healthcare providers, the healthcare system, and third-party payors; provide information to assist in informed decision-making; and support decisions that a patient makes.

The home health nurse also:

- Identifies and coordinates community resources to assist patients in achieving optimal health potential

- Empowers patients and families in their interactions with the healthcare system by providing information and support

- Provides information about care options, costs of care, reimbursement systems, and community resources to advocate for and support patient choice

- Implements programs, such as medication reconciliation and fall prevention, to maximize patient safety

- Refers the patient to community services and resources to ensure continuity of care after discharge from home care

- Promotes continuity of care through collaboration within the agency and with other healthcare providers

Administrative Roles

ADMINISTRATOR

The home health nurse administrator assumes a leadership role and is responsible for maintaining quality care in a dynamic environment in which reimbursement requirements, accreditation standards, and healthcare systems change frequently. The administrator provides leadership to meet these challenges and ensures availability of competent, qualified staff. The administrator must be knowledgeable about technologies, financial issues, documentation, and new opportunities while maintaining organizational and patient care standards. As the conscience of the organization, the administrator defines the values and concentrates on the mission of the organization and its first priority: namely, the patient and the patient's needs (Harris, 2010). The administrator who serves in this dynamic, multifaceted role also:

- Serves as a liaison between staff and outside agencies, including national and legal entities

- Speaks for home health staff and patients and brings attention to problems and limitations of the present system

- Creates an environment that facilitates and encourages nursing staff to demonstrate accountability for their own practice

- Establishes an environment that gives nurses a voice in the decision-making process

- Shapes the environment in which nurses practice and teach and consumers receive evidence-based home health care

- Creates a service-oriented environment in which high-quality health care services are emphasized to meet or exceed the needs of internal and external customers

- Utilizes professional skills such as decision-making, creativity, innovation, and communication to establish policies, procedures, and programs to accomplish goals

- Establishes cost-effective budgets and strategies using strategies that include analyzing and controlling variances to maintain expenses within approved limits

- Evaluates agency programs, performance, efficacy, effectiveness, and efficiency, and works with stakeholders to set future goals

- Assesses community needs to determine opportunities to develop programs to meet the needs of the community/population

- Establishes partnerships with other community groups to fill gaps and expand services to patients and families

- Formulates policies and procedures that reflect current practice in order to comply with federal, state, and other regulatory standards

SUPERVISOR OR CLINICAL MANAGER

The home health supervisor or clinical manager is responsible and accountable for organizing, coordinating, and evaluating the clinical practice activities. This individual oversees programs for the provision of nursing services to patients of all ages in the community and manages nursing practice to ensure adherence to standards and procedures. The nurse in this role also:

- Reviews intake data and assures safe transition processes

- Oversees the delivery of patient care on a daily basis

- Facilitates the professional development of home health nurses by providing education and support in clinical decision-making and disease management

- Assures compliance with regulations related to certification, accreditation, and the organization in the care delivery process

- Supports achievement of the organization's mission and goals by ensuring the availability of competent nursing staff

- Evaluates the professional performance of nursing staff

- Performs annual employee appraisals to ensure compliance with internal and external standards

- Manages and guides home care nurses to ensure the provision of quality patient care

- Evaluates clinical documentation to ensure compliance with organization, accreditation, certification, and state nurse practice acts.

- Interviews professional nurses to ensure the hiring of qualified staff

- Communicates information both verbally and in writing in a timely, clear, and concise manner
- Maintains an understanding of home health regulations to ensure appropriate reimbursement for services

QUALITY AND PERFORMANCE IMPROVEMENT NURSE

The nurse leader who is responsible for quality and performance improvement promotes excellence in clinical practice in the organization. This is accomplished by assessing, planning, organizing, administering, and coordinating all aspects of the program. This individual:

- Plans, implements, and evaluates the performance improvement program to ensure compliance with certification and accreditation requirements
- Collects and analyzes quantitative and qualitative data to evaluate patients' responses to care
- Tracks and trends data to determine positive outcome achievement and define opportunities for improvement
- Evaluates the organization's processes and structure to ensure that quality care is consistently delivered in the organization and determines when process redesign is needed
- Incorporates evidence-based practice into policies, procedures, and practices
- Provides education, support, and mentoring for new staff or supervisors
- Translates and disseminates quality data to appropriate stakeholders
- Communicates information both verbally and in writing, in a timely, clear, and concise manner to facilitate the organization's operation and meet reporting requirements

CLINICAL EDUCATOR

The clinical educator assumes a leadership position in a home health agency to facilitate the professional development of home health nurses and educate other staff on the organization's policies, procedures, and expectation. The home health clinical educator also:

- Assesses the learning needs and competence of staff to improve the level of performance, teaching skills, and quality of care, and assure compliance with accreditation standards

- Develops, implements, and evaluates continuing education programs for all levels of staff to ensure achievement of departmental and individual goals

- Plans, implements, and evaluates the orientation program to educate new staff on the agency's vision, mission, policies, procedures, and role expectations

- Participates in the development of competency standards for new or expanded clinical service programs

- Develops teaching tools and resources to facilitate patient education and understanding

- Collaborates with affiliating educational institutions to plan and arrange practicum experiences for students

This role also includes accountability for advocacy initiatives for both professional development and the professional practice of home health nursing. The responsibilities include ongoing education, mentoring, contributing to the ongoing development of the practice through active participation in professional membership, promoting the image of professional home health nursing, and actively participating in legislation and research that affect home health nursing. Other professional advocacy responsibilities include:

- Acting as a role model for professional nursing and as a proactive nursing advocate

- Supporting and encouraging others to study and practice nursing

- Sharing knowledge and experience with colleagues within and outside of home health

- Serving as a leader in health promotion and patient care by advancing one's own knowledge base

- Incorporating concepts of evidence-based practice in planning nursing interventions

- Fostering cohesive relationships and collaboration with all members of the nursing profession

- Maintaining membership and active involvement in professional organizations to remain current in health policy that impacts practice
- Participating in formal quality assessment and improvement activities

INFORMATICS LIAISON NURSE

The presence of nurse leaders demonstrating current technology skills and informatics knowledge has risen in importance in recent years due to federal requirements mandating implementation of electronic health records. Electronic documentation enhances patient safety and may also be the foundational vehicle for information sharing and collaboration across settings and care transitions. Effective and efficient documentation and information and technology management are crucial to success in meeting regulatory and accreditation standards and the data collection necessary for performance improvement.

The informatics liaison home health nurse works to integrate informatics science within the practice of home health by performing these functions:

- Exhibiting extensive experience in home health so as to be able to guide staff in searching out key safety information in the record
- Teaching staff to document a comprehensive assessment, develop a plan of care, and measure patient success toward outcome achievement
- Determining staff competency to complete clear, accurate documentation
- Partnering with leadership to define reports needed to demonstrate safe care along with regulatory compliance and clinical outcome achievement
- Optimizing information management and communication among caregivers
- Serving as an agency representative and liaison with agency health information technology staff and the clinical team
- Serving as team leader for system selection criteria and liaison to external decision-making bodies for selection of vendors and agency information staff
- Addressing usability and regulatory issues related to mobile health (m-health) technologies and other implemented solutions

Trends, Issues, and Opportunities in Home Health Nursing

Home health nurses, their organizations, and the healthcare industry face dynamic, though challenging, trends, issues, and opportunities. Five areas are addressed in this section: practice environment, ethics, research, informatics and health technology, and finances and reimbursement. Woven throughout this section are comments about the need for home health nurses and their home health care agencies to:

- Acknowledge the volatile healthcare environment at the state and national levels

- Be proactive participants in the change process

- Advocate for quality home health nursing care while remaining mindful of the numerous practice and ethical issues that are encountered during the course of providing care to patients

- Increasingly contribute to and move forward with implementing best evidence-based practices

- Participate in research opportunities with the goal of improved patient outcomes

- Be trailblazers in the use of information technology to improve the quality of patient care

- Recognize financial challenges based on legislative and regulatory changes that impact patient care and reimbursement for home health care services

- Develop strategic plans to avoid a negative impact on patient care and agency viability

- Embrace interprofessional collaboration

The following subsections deal with trends, issues, and opportunities that influence the role of today's home health nurse and are likely to do so even more during the next few years.

Practice Environments

The ability of nurses to provide compassionate and effective care is as dependent on the environment in which nurses practice as it is upon their knowledge, skills, abilities, and attitudes. The homes and communities in which home health nurses work are one element of their practice environment. The practice environment of home health nurses includes the milieu in which nurses work: the pressures, benefits, and opportunities that affect their lives. This environment should be safe and personally and professionally rewarding for the home health nurse. Safety issues that should be addressed with home health care clinicians were identified by NIHSH (2010); they included identifying/dealing with dangerous/abusive situations, ergonomics, latex allergies, infection prevention, presence of personal protective equipment, dealing with animals, and safe driving practices (NIHSH, 2010).

Over the next years, several pressures may have a negative impact on home health nurses' practice environment, unless home health nurses recognize and respond to them as opportunities. These pressures include the structural and financial uncertainties of healthcare reform, the impact of accountable care organizations (ACOs), and the effect of pay-for-quality performance initiatives. The demographics of an aging population and projections of nursing shortages add additional pressures to an already fragile environment. At the same time, agencies need to invest in, and nurses need to master, the ever more technologically advanced care devices, health information, documentation, and communication systems.

Home health agencies will be hard pressed to meet shifting financial demands. As a result, nurses providing care to patients in the patients' homes will likely be expected to be increasingly more productive and efficient at providing care while simultaneously enhancing patient outcomes. Home health nurses must be vigilant in ensuring that agency short-term financial goals contribute to positive practice environments and are not achieved at the expense of patient care goals and expected outcomes.

Agencies need to attract and retain highly skilled and motivated nurses if they intend to achieve the quality patient outcomes that home health agencies desire and patients and their families expect. Home health nurses must help their agencies create positive practice environments. ANCC's *Magnet Recognition Program* (http://www.nursecredentialing.org/Magnet.aspx) has identified factors in the practice environment that lead to nursing excellence and quality patient outcomes. Similarly, based upon nursing literature, research, and expert opinion, ANCC's *Pathway to Excellence Program* (http://www.nursecredentialing.org/Pathway) has identified standards that characterize healthcare organizations committed to the type of positive practice environments highly valued by nurses, including home health nurses. Using the

Magnet and Pathway standards as a foundation, home health nurses should advocate within their agencies for the following changes to create a positive work environment.

Practice environments that attract nurses include ones where excellent nursing practice is expected and supported. Excellent nursing practice includes agency expectations for high ethical and professional standards for patient care. Nurses should help shape agency standards, voice concerns, and develop solutions to problems that affect their patients and their working environment through shared governance.

A positive practice environment includes appropriate compensation and benefits that are competitive with other practice settings and with which nurses can support their families. Staffing levels should not overburden nurses with productivity requirements that compromise their ability to provide quality care or maintain work-life balance. Nurses should advocate for safe work environments. For example, sharps safety devices should be standard, and nurses should advocate for devices that support safe patient lifting, handling, and mobility to protect patients, themselves, home health aides, and other care providers, including family members, from musculoskeletal injuries (ANA, 2013b).

Because home health nurses practice alone in the community, they are subject to many hazardous situations not encountered by nurses in more controlled settings. Risks of driving to patients' homes in inclement weather, visiting patients in dangerous or violent neighborhoods, working in homes that present undue hazards, and admitting patients or families or caregivers who may be dangerous or violent can put nurses' personal safety at risk (NIHSH, 2010). Many times home health nurses are the ones who can best evaluate the risk because only they are "at the scene."

Thus, home health nurses should participate in developing organizational policies and procedures, using recommendations from the nursing and safety literature, to protect themselves and their colleagues from violence or injury. They must have the autonomy and authority to decide which patients, families, caregivers, homes, or neighborhoods unduly expose them and their colleagues to such risks. Home health nurses should not do anything that puts their health or safety at undue risk. At times, leaving the patient's home immediately is the best way of securing the nurse's safety. Once the nurse is safe, alternate plans can be developed to meet the patient's needs.

Nurses are drawn to organizations that support career ladders, continuing education, certification, pursuit of academic degrees, and involvement in professional and specialty nursing organizations. Nurses should advocate for orientation and staff development programs that enable them to feel appropriately prepared for the care their patients need. Nurses should advocate for their home health agencies to recognize nurse achievement, experience, and expertise by supporting clinical ladder programs, specialty certification, academic degrees, and nursing organization participation. This must include financial support: Home health nurses are an investment in quality patient care and better outcomes, which ultimately assure agency sustainability.

The ability to provide both evidence-based care and patient-centered care is part of a positive practice environment. Because scientific studies are being published at an increasingly rapid pace, to keep their practice congruent with current evidence, home health nurses need access to clinical literature, databases, and guidelines that assimilate research into standards for evidence-based practice. They also need access to clinical nurse specialists and other advanced practice registered nurses who are experts in helping clinicians and agencies incorporate evidence into practice.

Although evidence-based care is foundational to quality nursing care, nurses must also advocate for the ability to practice patient-centered care: patient-centered care demands that nurses identify, understand, and care about their patients' individual needs and preferences, and then adapt that care to meet those needs and preferences. This enables patients to feel valued and respected, a particularly important outcome in today's ever more culturally diverse population. At times, patient-centered care will require nurses to individualize the care they derive from care pathways and evidence-based guidelines to meet patient needs and preferences.

Patient-centered care uses evidence-based patient engagement strategies. These strategies motivate patients to become more actively engaged partners in monitoring their own health status and adhering to the treatment plans that promote their health. Patient engagement interventions include motivational interviewing, breaking long-term goals into action plans with SMART (specific, measurable, achievable, relevant, time-defined) goals that foster patient success, and "zone tools" for monitoring health status. Home health nurses use adult learning, health literacy, coaching, positive reinforcement, problem-solving, and information-sharing principles when providing patient education (VNAA, 2013).

Many factors coalesce to form a positive practice environment for home health nurses. Home health nurses cannot be passive participants in their practice environment, but must help build a practice environment that attracts other highly motivated and skilled nurses into home health nursing. During this period of healthcare reform, home health nurses should seize the opportunity to help develop positive practice environments.

Ethics in Home Health Nursing

Situations requiring ethical decision-making are ubiquitous in home health nursing. Faced with designing and implementing a plan of care that is, by nature of the practice setting, collaborative with the patient, family, and other caregivers, nurses find that decisions regarding *how* care is delivered are complex and influenced by the values, health beliefs, culture, religion, prognosis, finances, capabilities, and motivations of both patient and family/other caregivers. Home health nurses must be comfortable with and confident in their listening and negotiating skills to actually extract the patient's desires and intentions about care while being able to respect the patient's autonomy and perform within professional boundaries. The nine provisions of *Code of Ethics for Nurses with Interpretive Statements* (ANA, 2001) provide a guiding framework for ethical nursing practice in home health.

RESPECT FOR THE INDIVIDUAL

Provision 1. The nurse, in all professional relationships, practices with compassion and respect for the inherent dignity, worth, and uniqueness of every individual, unrestricted by considerations of social or economic status, personal attributes, or the nature of health problems.

Respecting patient autonomy is especially challenging when the patient's desires collide with apparent safety needs. Caregiver abilities may be less than capable or financial resources inadequate, and yet the patient is determined to "remain at home," even when this plan is considered unsafe by others. The home health nurse must astutely, yet respectfully, extract the objective data during visits and read "between the visits" to facilitate the patient's reaching a safer decision or vigorously obtain as many resources as possible from the community that will enable the patient to remain at home while benefiting from care.

COMMITMENT TO THE PATIENT

Provision 2. The nurse's primary commitment is to the patient, whether an individual, family, group, or community.

Patients who do not adhere to the prescribed plan of care should not be labeled "noncompliant." Research indicates that nonadherence occurs due to many factors, such as low literacy, low self-esteem, and subtle cognitive impairment. This demands that nurses provide expert comprehensive assessment, interviewing, counseling, educating, and coaching skills to assist patients to a higher level of wellness, thereby avoiding rehospitalization. The skills that these patients need, however, can take time that affects adequate agency reimbursement. Third-party payors may question the appropriateness of the extended lengths of stay these patients require to achieve improved outcomes. The question "Is the patient benefiting from home health care?" (or the opposing side, "Would discharge harm this patient?") must be carefully weighed and balanced on ethical principles of beneficence, nonmaleficence, and distributive justice.

End-of-life discussions may be particularly difficult conversations. Yet, ethical practice requires home health nurses to help the patient and family learn about the various treatment options, possible trajectories, and outcomes, all presented in an unbiased way. These conversations, which often occur in the middle of a busy day while other patients wait for scheduled visits, can be as stressful for the nurse as they are for the patient. Such conversations demand the nurse's time, focus, and sensitivity to elicit and advocate for the patient's desires.

ADVOCACY FOR THE PATIENT

Provision 3. The nurse promotes, advocates for, and strives to protect the health, safety, and rights of the patient.

This provision must be integral to every home health nurse's practice. Privacy issues may be difficult to negotiate when the patient depends on a partner or adult children for obtaining food, medications, supplies, and equipment, and for physical care. Privacy must also be protected within the community when the nurse also provides care to neighbors. Protecting patient privacy requires extra attention and care while answering cell phones and using paper and electronic documentation systems and other technologies within the community.

RESPONSIBILITY AND ACCOUNTABILITY FOR PRACTICE

Provision 4. The nurse is responsible and accountable for individual nursing practice and determines the appropriate delegation of tasks consistent with the nurse's obligation to provide optimum patient care.

The home health nurse is responsible for implementation of the patient's plan of care. In the home health setting, caregivers of various skill levels frequently work alone with the patient. It is the home health nurse's judgment that determines the care team members needed for a specific patient, based on that individual's needs. When delegating care plan tasks to unlicensed caregivers, such as home health aides, it is paramount that the home health nurse understand not only the patient's needs, but also the competency level of the specific aide. Such an assessment may require the home health nurse to instruct and supervise, to ensure that the patient receives safe, quality care.

DUTIES TO SELF AND OTHERS

Provision 5. The nurse owes the same duties to self as to others, including the responsibility to preserve integrity and safety, to maintain competence, and to continue personal and professional growth.

The home health nurse must be fully engaged in lifelong learning to maintain competence in the challenging and complex environment of home health services. (See Standard 8, Education, for more details.) Regulatory and reporting mandates change very frequently and often require significant interpretive skills and clinician knowledge. Maintenance of personal health and safety parameters permit home health nurses to counter the stresses associated with providing health care with limited or nonexistent resources.

CONTRIBUTIONS TO HEALTHCARE ENVIRONMENTS

Provision 6. The nurse participates in establishing, maintaining, and improving healthcare environments and conditions of employment conducive to the provision of quality health care and consistent with the values of the profession through individual and collective action.

Nursing leaders have a responsibility to support and provide resources for their staff. Leaders should employ education, case conferences, and ethics committee discussions to support appropriate decision-making that is within professional boundaries. In addition, leaders and staff may be called upon to help acquire necessary resources for patients and families. With the demands of staff productivity and oversight of publicly reported outcomes, home health managers are challenged to provide such supportive activities to staff and still regulate themselves through a collegial process of peer review of practice. Justice and implementation of a just work culture require home health managers and supervisors to redesign management processes to be most effective for both patients and staff.

ADVANCEMENT OF THE NURSING PROFESSION

Provision 7. The nurse participates in the advancement of the profession through contributions to practice, education, administration, and knowledge development.

Practice, education, administration, and knowledge development are intertwined and each contributes to professional nursing. Administration needs to establish and maintain an environment where nurses can incorporate research and evidence-based practice for safe and effective patient care. Home health care educators need to introduce and implement ANA nursing standards during orientation and continuing education programs to support the ongoing needs of nurses. This requires awareness of existing standards, participation in establishment of new and updated standards, and creation of new knowledge that individual nurses incorporate into daily nursing care to benefit patients. Nurses need to hold themselves and colleagues accountable for the care patients receive. Pursuing additional education, continuing education, reading journals, serving as preceptors, and being respectful of colleagues and students are ways to achieve the aims of this provision.

COLLABORATION TO MEET HEALTH NEEDS

Provision 8. The nurse collaborates with other health professionals and the public in promoting community, national, and international efforts to meet health needs.

Collaboration with other health professionals is a core part of the everyday work for a home health nurse. At the start of home care, the home health nurse assesses the patient and collaborates with the physician to design a plan of care designed specifically to move the patient toward optimal outcomes, supported by all needed disciplines, including physical, occupational, speech, and behavioral/mental health therapies, social work, and a home health aide as needed. This plan of care is periodically revised through the case conferencing of the care team.

By the nature of work in the community, the home health nurse participates in educating individuals and groups regarding numerous health topics. Case finding and referrals to health care are also common through participation in community health screenings and work with other groups. National efforts include home health nurses participating in quality standards setting, promoting efforts that enhance access to care, and collaborating with other health care professionals in research that supports health issues internationally.

PROMOTION OF THE NURSING PROFESSION

Provision 9. The profession of nursing, as represented by associations and their members, is responsible for articulating nursing values, for maintaining the integrity of the profession and its practice, and for shaping social policy.

Home health nurses join other home health leaders in countering the reduction of reimbursement for care. Much pressure is placed on agencies to provide more efficient care with fewer resources. Leaders may find themselves having to make challenging decisions regarding types of patients to serve, correct coding of episodes of care, and assessment data that could affect reimbursement. Some may be asked to deny care or provide care in less-than-effective ways for budgetary reasons that do not coincide with their values.

Nurse leaders must embrace strong ethical principles as they address the challenges of agency administration, establish partnerships with other healthcare institutions, and balance these actions with the principle of "do no harm." They carefully manage resources to consistently provide excellent patient and community care while simultaneously complying with regulations and reimbursement rules.

Research in Home Health Nursing

Diverse research that is pertinent to home health nursing practice includes case studies, studies conducted by members of other disciplines or interdisciplinary teams involving home health nurses, and programs of research. In general, the number of home health nurse researchers and the extent of funded home health studies remain small, especially in comparison to acute and long-term care research. The degree of rigor of the home health studies varies.

In 2005, a Delphi study was published that identified research priorities for home health care; these priorities included outcomes, health policy, the use of advanced practice nurses, and models of care and best practice (Madigan & Vanderboom, 2005). There has not been another study of home health research priorities since that date. This section gives a brief overview highlighting some key areas of clinical research and research programs.

The Centers for Medicare & Medicaid Services identified reduction of the hospitalization rate of home health patients as a national priority. This emphasis has stimulated research on patient risk factors related to home care and interventions and strategies to reduce such risks. A survey of home health agencies with the lowest hospitalization rates (Briggs Corporation, 2006;

NAHC, 2006) identified 15 agency strategies as instrumental in preventing hospitalizations; these strategies included assessing and reducing the risks for falls, increasing home visit frequency at the start of care, and giving attention to organizational culture.

Although most research related to adverse events has focused on inpatient settings, an understanding of adverse events in the home health setting is necessary to address patient safety. In a "scoping" review of the home care literature, categories of adverse events included adverse events related to medications, intravenous lines, technology issues and failures, infections, urinary catheters, wounds, and falls (Masotti, McColl, & Green, 2010). The researchers stress the need to study interventions that reduce the risk of adverse outcomes.

Preventing rehospitalization among home care patients remains a challenge. Patients with heart failure and rehospitalizations have perhaps been the most studied. Because optimal interventions in hospitalization prevention remain unclear, both health-care-specific interventions and healthcare policy must be examined (Madigan, Gordon, Fortinsky, Koroukian, Piña, & Riggs, 2012). Some success in reducing the risk of rehospitalization has been achieved with the use of telemonitoring systems as a tool, as addressed in the following section.

Other research has focused on fall risk identification, impact of falls, and interventions (e.g., Spoelstra, Given, You, & Given, 2012; Calys, Gagnon, & Jernigan, 2012; Monsen, Westra, Oancea, Yu, & Kerr, 2011). Medication management is a challenge as the patient transitions from one health care setting to another; medication discrepancies between hospital and home were found to be alarmingly high in one study (Corbett, Setter, Daratha, Nuemiller, & Wood, 2010). Strategies to improve patient self-care management, including nurse coaching, are being studied and were found to improve outcomes for patients with chronic conditions (Vincent & Birkhead, 2013).

Infection prevention is a growing concern in home health care, because infections contribute to morbidity, mortality, and increased cost of care. In a recent study, approximately 12% of home health patients had an infection, the most common being urinary tract infections, pneumonia, and cellulitis (Dwyer et al., 2013). In 2007, the Centers for Disease Control and Prevention (CDC) (Siegel, Rhinehart, Jackson, & Chiarello, 2007) published the first practice guideline incorporating recommendations aimed at prevention of multidrug-resistant organism infections that specifically addressed the home health setting. In 2008, the Association for Professionals in Infection Control and Epidemiology (APIC) and the CDC's Healthcare Infection Control Practices Advisory Committee (HICPAC) (APIC et al., 2008) published infection surveillance definitions for home health that asserted the importance of safety and quality of care in infection prevention. There is an urgent need to identify infections and to identify best practices for the home care setting aimed at reducing them.

Due to population demographics and the prevalence of chronic illnesses among home care patients, there is a growing focus on providing palliative home care. A Cochrane review of 23 studies evaluating the impact of palliative care found that home palliative care services increased the chances of the patient dying at home (the desire of most people), reduced symptom burden, and did not have an impact on caregiver grief (Gomes, Calanzani, Curiale, McCrone, & Higginson, 2013). Furthermore, hospice care provided in the home setting is associated with a general reduction in health care use and enhanced patient and family satisfaction (Candy, Holman, Leurent, Davis, & Jones, 2011).

Evidence-based practice and evidence-based guidelines are important to home health nurses. Clinical practice guidelines developed by the University of Iowa School of Nursing (e.g., gerontological interventions), the American Heart Association/American College of Cardiology (e.g., guidelines for heart failure management), the CDC (as identified earlier), and the Infusion Nurses Society (e.g., standards for infusion device care and infusion administration) are examples of such efforts. Although the number of studies specific to home health and capable of serving as a foundation for evidence-based home health practice remains relatively small, increasing interest encourages expansion of the research base, increased opportunities for home health nurse researchers, more interdisciplinary collaboration, improved funding, and better client outcomes.

Programs of clinical and administrative research offer the greatest opportunities for continuation and expansion. The following are examples of ongoing research programs that reflect the chronology of evidence-based research and best practices in home health.

Omaha System: The Omaha System is one of the 12 classification systems or standardized terminologies recognized by ANA. Four federally funded studies were conducted between 1975 and 1993 to develop and refine the Omaha System and to establish reliability, validity, and usability. The research led to use of standardized assessment, intervention, and outcomes management in practice sites nationally and globally, and integration of the Omaha System into software; it also stimulated further research. In 2005, more than 50 unique studies were organized into 8 categories and summarized; those studies were conducted by clinicians, managers, educators, students, and researchers (Martin, 2005; Monsen & Kerr, 2004). In 2013, 56 new Omaha System research publications were summarized; the goal was to evaluate the methodological quality of the studies, identify major trends, and suggest future research (Topaz, Golfenshtein, & Bowles, 2014). The authors noted two important trends. First, they described the shift from a focus on health-related problems of study subjects to an aggregate approach involving outcomes, classification, and interoperability research. Second, they described the increasing body of international literature. Most studies have been published in journals, books, or online (Omaha System, 2013). Two examples that incorporate practice, outcomes management, and electronic health records were published by Westra et al. (2011) and Plemmons et al. (Plemmons, Lipton, Fong, & Acosta, 2012).

Transitional care: In 1989, Naylor et al. began to study high-risk elders and the discharge planning process (Naylor, Stephens, Bowles, & Bixby, 2005). At the University of Pennsylvania, the Transitional Care Model (TCM) has been developed and refined over the past 20 years. The TCM includes the components of a master's prepared nurse, comprehensive assessment, and interdisciplinary coordination (including home visits). Outcomes include reduced hospitalizations and healthcare costs and short-term improvements in health-related outcomes (Transitional Care Model, n.d.; Naylor et al., 2011).

Outcome and Assessment Information Set (OASIS): In the United States, OASIS data are used for home health regulation, reimbursement, clinical purposes, and research. OASIS data have been used to analyze and evaluate home health clinical outcomes, including outcomes for wound healing, home health service use, and adverse events among home health patients. Debate over the validity and reliability of OASIS continue. In a systematic literature review, study results were found to be tentative and additional research was called for to validate the OASIS tool in measurement of patient outcomes, in research, and in quality improvement (O'Connor & Davitt, 2012). In a large retrospective cohort study, several elements of OASIS data were found useful in identifying patients at risk for pressure ulcers (Bergquist-Beringer & Gajewski, 2011).

The Visiting Nurse Service (VNS) of New York: In 1994, a home health research center was established. Its sound research and practice improvement initiative have enabled it to attract major grants from private philanthropists and government funding agencies and increasingly to work collaboratively with the home health industry, academic institutions, and quality improvement organizations to improve home care. The center's research focuses on four main areas: improving the quality and outcomes of home health services; helping persons to better manage chronic conditions; analyzing and informing public policies that affect home-based care and access to long-term care; and supporting communities that promote successful aging in place (VNS of New York, 2013).

Informatics in Home Health Nursing

Technology and information technology are tools that can improve the public's health (Friedman, Parrish, & Ross, 2013; Nelson & Staggers, 2014). These tools are evolving rapidly both in this country and globally, influencing the practice of home health nurses and transforming home health agency operations. Historically, home health nurses, their clinician colleagues, and their agencies have been innovators and early adopters of diverse communication devices and technology (Rogers, 1995). Increasingly, nurses, their agencies, and their patients are embracing mobile phones, fall detection devices, information systems, electronic health records, personal health records, the Internet, and telemonitoring. They often consider these necessities (Suter & Hennessey, 2011; Martin & Utterback, 2014).

Patients and their families frequently use the Internet to become informed about diagnoses, medications, and treatments, and to exchange information with others. They use personal alarm systems and various devices to increase their safety and monitor their health status. Home health agencies are investing in more sophisticated hardware, software, and telemonitoring equipment due to improved selection, changes in Medicare regulations and reimbursement, and market demand. Two major trends, telemonitoring and electronic health records (EHRs), are the focus of this section.

Many home health agencies use a technology referred to as *telehealth*, *telemonitoring*, or *remote patient monitoring*. The Veterans Administration has also incorporated this technology into many of its programs. *Telehealth* is "the use of electronic information and telecommunications technologies to support long-distance clinical health care, patient and professional health-related education, public health, and health administration" (U.S. Department of Health and Human Services [U.S. DHHS], 2013).

Telehealth within the framework of home health nursing can be broadly defined as the delivery of patient care services using technology to eliminate distance, time, or resource barriers in an effort to improve patient health outcomes. The goal of telemonitoring is to increase the effectiveness and efficiency of communication, so as to achieve enhanced quality of care, improved patient and clinician safety, and increased productivity (Madigan et al., 2013; Schlachta-Fairchild et al., 2014). Woods and Snow (2013) conducted a study in a home health agency with patients who had circulatory and/or respiratory diagnoses; patients who participated in a telemonitoring intervention had significantly lower rates of rehospitalization and emergency room use. Hoban et al. (Hoban, Fedor, Reeder, & Chernick, 2013) studied patients with heart failure and found that those who were monitored were more likely to adopt self-care behaviors to ensure their well-being. Another study focused on patients who transitioned from the hospital to home, had heart failure, and used telemonitoring; findings from this pilot study included improved communication and no hospital readmissions (Heeke, Wood, & Schuck, 2014).

Telemonitoring applications include, but are not limited to, the following:

- Telemonitors with peripheral biometric attachments for remotely monitoring biophysical parameters such as weight, or more complex measurements such as oxygen saturation or glucose levels.

- Phone technology with two-way connectivity that allows monitoring of patient activity or response to disease management parameters such as pain, activity level, symptom exacerbation, diet, or behavioral cues. This information may be correlated with biophysical parameters.

- In-home message devices with disease management education, advice, and medication or treatment reminders, with compliance monitoring features that may be remotely transmitted via phone or Internet technology or evaluated at nursing visits.

- Video cameras for monitoring all aspects of care delivery; uses have focused particularly on wound management, home care aide supervision, and other aspects of clinical care usually necessitating direct observation.

- Personal computers with Internet connectivity for supervised communication, medical record access, or patient education.

- Videoconferencing that allows nurses, physicians, and other healthcare providers to communicate about patient-specific care or to learn new disease management interventions.

Information systems, electronic health records (EHRs), and electronic personal health records (PHRs) are becoming ubiquitous. According to a 2009 survey (Fazzi Associates, 2009), approximately 65% of reporting home health agencies had EHRs. In a 2013 survey (Fazzi Associates, 2013), approximately 77% of reporting agencies had EHRs. The percentages increased even more in office-based physician practices and hospitals because of the financial incentives offered by the Office of the National Coordinator's meaningful-use implementation strategies. In physician practices, EHR use increased from approximately 48% in 2009 to 72% in 2012 (CDC, 2012). The percentage of use in hospitals more than doubled in the past few years, increasing from 16% in 2009 to 35% in 2011 (*Medical News Today*, 2012). However, such increases unfortunately do not represent an enhanced capacity to collaborate and exchange patient data, especially with regard to transitions of care between providers and settings.

An EHR is a longitudinal collection of a patient's health-related information stored in a computer-readable format. A PHR is also an electronic collection of health-related information, but it is managed and controlled by the individual. Federal mandates and incentives have promoted use of these resources. Beginning with executive orders in 2004, the federal government established the Office of the National Coordinator for Health Information Technology (http://www.hhs.gov/healthit), the agenda of which proposes that all documentation be converted to electronic systems in the near future. The Health Information Technology for Economic and Clinical Health (HITECH) Act of 2009 created the term *meaningful use*, and added details about health information technology (Blumenthal & Tavenner, 2010; Friedman, Parrish, & Ross, 2013). The "Triple Aim" has evolved from these efforts, with national goals to (1) improve health care quality and experience, (2) improve the health of populations, and (3) reduce the per capita cost of health care (adapted from Berwick, Nolan, & Whittington, 2008).

Many home health agencies are investing in robust clinical, financial, scheduling, and statistical management information systems that are patient-centered and evidence-based; some are more integrated than those of their local hospitals (Martin, 2005; Bowles et al., 2013; Hall, Poole, & Hall, 2013; Nelson & Staggers, 2014). EHRs are the foundation of these systems. Potential home health benefits include improving the quality of care and practice, ranging from care involving one patient and one clinician to care by the entire agency and to the entire population, which are benefits closely aligned with the Triple Aim.

Standardization and standardized terminologies are required before the full range of EHR benefits can be realized across all settings. The two types of standardized terminologies are:

- Standardized point-of-care or interface terminology: a structured language consisting of terms, definitions, and codes that clinicians use to guide and document practice

- Standardized reference terminology: a structured language consisting of terms, definitions, and codes that clinicians do not see, but software developers use to promote interoperability.

The Omaha System is an example of a standardized point-of-care terminology used by many home health agencies. The three components of the Omaha System integrate assessment, interventions, and outcomes management (Martin, 2005). Other point-of-care terminologies recognized by ANA include Clinical Care Classification, North American Nursing Diagnosis Association (NANDA) International, Nursing Interventions Classification (NIC), and Nursing Outcomes Classification (NOC) (ANA, 2013a). SNOMED CT®, LOINC®, and HL7 are reference terminologies and were selected as the national standards to increase interoperability. The goal is for providers to be linked and patients' clinical data to be exchanged in a secure environment.

Without standardization, use of best practices, clinical decision support systems, care coordination, interprofessional communication, outcomes management, interoperability, and exchange of data, health information exchanges (HIE) and accountable care organizations (ACOs) are limited. Bowles et al. (2013) identified serious challenges when attempting to implement a decision support system and conduct research in four hospitals that used the same EHR. The standardization challenges involved limited documentation policies and quality improvement programs, customization, and user interface. Home care agencies and nurses encounter similar information exchange and transition issues.

The trend to adopt models of care, standardized terminologies, EHRs, the Internet, and information technology is a global, not a national, trend. The Netherlands is a leader in this movement (Monsen & deBlok, 2013). Individuals, groups, and countries with fewer economic resources than the United States are beginning to obtain and communicate health-related information by using mobile phones and other devices. Vendors are developing smaller and faster digital and multifunctional devices. Web access is expected to replace current technology, and web-based education is rapidly advancing.

Today's home health nurses will soon need to use new devices and methods that have yet to be invented. Similarly, their patients will use new technologies, including microchips, to store their personal health data. Home health nurses who anticipate and embrace technological developments as tools will experience many positive outcomes for their patients, their community, and the public's health.

Finances and Reimbursement

Topics related to finances and reimbursement in home health care include:

- Access to care
- Agency viability
- Patient outcomes vs. agency costs
- Technology costs
- Implementation of the new International Classification of Diseases coding system (ICD 10) and its significant impact on home health organizations and practice, as well as on legislation/health care reform
- Payment models, such as ACOs, medical homes, and value-based purchasing

In the United States, the Patient Protection and Affordable Care Act is challenging healthcare entities to provide quality care that is cost-effective. Other countries throughout the world are also facing reforms to their healthcare systems. Home health agencies must examine their practices and payor mix. Additionally, they must undertake strategic initiatives to remain viable and capable of participating in a healthcare system that is being reshaped and remodeled. The following is a list of projected trends:

Access. Patients will have increased access to care and will be increasingly responsible for sharing the cost of health care. Patients and families will have greater access to a variety of primary healthcare providers, increase their use of more advanced telemonitoring systems, and interact with a variety of accountable care organizations and medical home models and their services for enhanced continuity of care. Costs could possibly be prohibitive and cause patients to refuse home care visits.

Patient engagement. Patient accountability for self-care and autonomy will become increasingly important, as more emphasis will be placed on reduction of healthcare costs and greater responsibility placed on the patient for self-care in disease management. This challenges home health nurses to design new approaches or models of care.

Evidence-based practice. Home health agencies must continue to find cost-effective standards of care that yield positive outcomes. Agencies must employ best practices to reduce costs associated with rehospitalization and emergent care use. Home health agencies will be financially rewarded for their efforts in resource reduction and positive outcomes with multiple payor sources.

Patient and financial outcomes. Home health agency reports of patient outcomes will require better understanding of data collection and reporting, as well as the enhanced management of business and financial intelligence and the associated metrics used to analyze agency performance. Accurate analysis of data requires comprehensive reports that collate data in a manner that allows management to understand the balance of revenue and utilization, along with patient outcomes and satisfaction.

Technological improvements. Technology, through the use of smartphones, point-of-care devices, and tablet applications, will allow healthcare providers, home health agencies, and patients to be more aware of personal health data trends. This will enable them to react quickly to changes in health status, thus providing interventions that may be less costly to the system and to the patient. Additionally, agency viability depends upon investment in the right information technology for access to the necessary business and financial information.

Regulatory requirements. Agencies must continually invest in their employees and provide education regarding coding, data collection, billing practices, and ongoing regulatory changes. Practice management systems must be able to accommodate ICD-10 if they are to meet regulatory compliance and accommodate newly developed diagnoses and procedures. Unless an agency invests in its people, to keep them up to date with the ever-changing environment, both the agency and its staff will suffer financially (www.cms.gov).

Home health nurses will be providing care through agencies that must continually evaluate their resources to find effective and efficient business models for viability within the reformed heath care system. The home health nurse must be aware of the ongoing changes to reimbursement/payment structures, keep up to date with technology, and remain a good steward of the resources provided to care for patients in the home.

Summary of the Scope of Home Health Nursing Practice

Home health nurses provide care in an ever-changing healthcare environment and will be at the forefront of the impending cataclysmic changes in health care. They provide skilled care in the home that was neither available nor anticipated even a few years ago. Expert assessment, clinical decision-making skills, and evidence-based practice, combined with a positive attitude and the willingness and ability to adapt to the constantly changing healthcare environment and related challenges, will help patients achieve optimal outcomes.

As more patients are cared for at home, care coordination and management will be key requisites in the home health nurse's repertoire and skill set. Those who practiced in home care during the difficult years of the interim payment system (IPS) and prospective payment system (PPS) will be applying knowledge gleaned from those experiences as they lead others through the current healthcare evolution. Estimates vary widely, but it is reasonable certain that many home care organizations as known today will cease to exist in the coming years.

Home health services will be more important than ever in the changing healthcare delivery model, but rendering these services effectively will take leadership, innovation, and risk-taking. Home health nurses must embrace change, adapt to external forces and changed payment models and other policies, and seize this opportunity to define and lead a new and more effective world of home care. Home health nurses will continue to be called upon to coordinate and deliver excellent care according to the highest standards. This updated scope of practice statement and revised standards of home health nursing practice are meant to guide, define, and direct home health professional nursing practice today as well as in the future.

Standards of Home Health Nursing Practice

Significance of the Standards

The *Standards of Professional Nursing Practice*, on which the Standards of Home Health Nursing Practice are based, are authoritative statements of the duties that all registered nurses, regardless of role, population, or specialty, are expected to perform competently. The standards published herein may be utilized as evidence of the standard of care, with the understanding that application of the standards is context dependent. The standards are subject to change with the dynamics of the nursing profession, as new patterns of professional practice are developed and accepted by the nursing profession and the public. In addition, specific conditions and clinical circumstances may affect the application of the standards at a given time (e.g., during a natural disaster). The standards are subject to formal, periodic review and revision.

The competencies that accompany each standard may be evidence of compliance with the corresponding standard. The list of competencies is not exhaustive. Whether a particular standard or competency applies depends on the circumstances.

Standards of Practice for Home Health Nursing

Standard 1. Assessment

The home health registered nurse collects comprehensive data pertinent to the patient's health and/or the situation.

COMPETENCIES
The home health registered nurse:

- Collects comprehensive data, including but not limited to physical, functional, nutrition, psychosocial, emotional, cognitive, sexual, cultural, age-related, environmental, spiritual/transpersonal, and economic assessments, in a systematic and ongoing process while honoring the uniqueness of the patient, family, and other caregivers.

- Elicits the patient's health beliefs, values, preferences, expressed needs, goals, and self-care behaviors, and knowledge of her or his healthcare situation.

- Obtains an accurate medication history and identifies medication discrepancies.

- Identifies deficits and barriers to effective performance of self-care management skills/behaviors.

- Involves the patient, family, other caregivers, and other healthcare providers in holistic data collection.

- Identifies barriers (e.g., psychosocial, literacy, health literacy, financial, cultural) to effective communication and makes appropriate adaptations.

- Recognizes the influence of personal attitudes, values, and beliefs, and the need to remove any bias.

- Assesses family dynamics, coping and caregiving skills, knowledge, and impact on patient health and wellness.

- Prioritizes data collection based on the patient's immediate condition and the anticipated needs of the patient, family, and other caregivers in the home.

- Uses appropriate evidence-based assessment techniques, instruments, and tools, such as falls risk assessments, nutritional assessment, pain scales, depression scales, and cognitive level measures.

- Synthesizes available data, information, and knowledge relevant to the situation to identify patterns and variances.

- Applies ethical, legal, and privacy guidelines and policies to the collection, maintenance, use, and dissemination of patient and other data and information.

- Recognizes patients as the authority on their own health by honoring their care preferences.

- Promotes sharing of assessment data through an electronic health record.

- Documents relevant assessment data in a retrievable format.

ADDITIONAL COMPETENCIES FOR THE GRADUATE-LEVEL PREPARED HOME HEALTH NURSE AND THE ADVANCED PRACTICE REGISTERED NURSE

The graduate-level prepared home health nurse or the advanced practice registered nurse:

- Initiates and interprets diagnostic tests and procedures relevant to the patient's current status.

- Uses known or innovative evidence-based assessment techniques and tools.

- Performs advanced assessments of home health patient populations with specific or complex needs.

- Assesses the effect of interactions among patients, family, caregivers, community, and social systems on health and illness.

STANDARDS OF HOME HEALTH NURSING PRACTICE

Standard 2. Diagnosis

The home health registered nurse analyzes the assessment data to determine the diagnoses, needs, or issues.

COMPETENCIES

The home health registered nurse:

- Derives the diagnoses, needs, or issues from assessment data.

- Validates the diagnoses, needs, or issues with the patient, family, other caregivers, and other healthcare providers.

- Identifies actual or potential risks to the patient's health and safety or barriers to health, which may include but are not limited to interpersonal, systematic, or environmental circumstances.

- Uses standardized classification systems and clinical decision support tools, when available, in identifying diagnoses.

- Documents diagnoses, needs, or issues in a manner that facilitates determination of the expected outcomes and plan.

ADDITIONAL COMPETENCIES FOR THE GRADUATE-LEVEL PREPARED HOME HEALTH NURSE AND THE ADVANCED PRACTICE REGISTERED NURSE

The graduate-level prepared home health nurse or the advanced practice registered nurse:

- Systematically compares and contrasts clinical findings with normal and abnormal variations and developmental events in formulating a differential diagnosis.

- Utilizes complex data and information obtained during interview, examination, and diagnostic processes in identifying diagnoses.

- Assists staff in developing and maintaining competence in the diagnostic process.

Standard 3. Outcomes Identification

The home health registered nurse identifies expected outcomes for a plan individualized to the patient, family, other caregivers, and caregiving situation.

COMPETENCIES

The home health registered nurse:

- Derives physical, psychosocial, and culturally appropriate expected outcomes from the diagnoses.

- Involves the patient, family, other caregivers, healthcare team members, and others in formulating expected outcomes.

- Collaborates with the patient to develop SMART goals (specific, measurable, achievable, relevant, and time-defined).

- Integrates the patient's goals when formulating expected outcomes.

- Considers associated risks, benefits, costs, potential barriers, current scientific evidence, and expected trajectory of the condition when formulating expected outcomes.

- Defines expected outcomes in terms of the patient's culture, values, and ethical beliefs.

- Includes a time estimate for the attainment of expected outcomes.

- Develops expected outcomes that support continuity of care.

- Modifies expected outcomes according to changes in the status of the patient, family, other caregivers, or home environment.

- Documents expected outcomes as measurable changes in the patient's status.

ADDITIONAL COMPETENCIES FOR THE GRADUATE-LEVEL PREPARED HOME HEALTH NURSE AND THE ADVANCED PRACTICE REGISTERED NURSE

The graduate-level prepared home health nurse or the advanced practice registered nurse:

- Identifies expected outcomes that incorporate scientific evidence and are achievable through implementation of evidence-based practices.

- Identifies expected outcomes that incorporate cost and clinical effectiveness, patient satisfaction, continuity, and consistency among providers.
- Differentiates outcomes that require care process interventions from those that require system-level interventions.
- Serves as a role model to staff investigating the latest evidence to support improvement of outcomes.
- Uses technology to incorporate evidence-based interventions and facilitate outcome achievement while engaging patients, families, and caregivers in the process.

Standard 4. Planning

The home health registered nurse develops a plan that prescribes strategies and alternatives to attain expected outcomes.

COMPETENCIES

The home health registered nurse:

- Collaborates with the patient, family, and other caregivers to develop an individualized plan that is adapted to the patient's unique needs and preferences, including, but not limited to:
  - Physical needs, comorbidities, and functional status.
  - Psychosocial needs, developmental level, health literacy, coping style, finances, and environment.
  - Spiritual and cultural values, beliefs, and health practices.
  - Available technologies and community-based resources.

- Includes strategies in the plan to address each of the patient's identified diagnoses, deficits, or issues. These strategies may include, but are not limited to, strategies for:
  - Promotion and restoration of health.
  - Prevention of illness, injury, and disease.
  - Alleviation of suffering.
  - Support of those who choose palliative care.

- Establishes the plan priorities with the patient, family, other caregivers, interprofessional team, and others involved with the patient's care.

- Integrates additional home health care or community-based services that help the patient meet the expected outcomes.

- Provides for smooth transitions to home care and on discharge from home care.

- Incorporates a timeline for expected outcomes within the plan.

- Considers the economic impact of the plan on the patient, family, other caregivers, agency, third-party payors, or other affected parties.

- Integrates best practices, research, and evidence-based practice guidelines into the plan.

- Defines the plan within the boundaries of current statutes, rules and regulations, and standards.

- Modifies the plan according to the ongoing assessment of the patient's response and feedback from family and caregivers, along with other outcome indicators.

- Documents the plan in a manner that uses standardized language or recognized terminology.

ADDITIONAL COMPETENCIES FOR THE GRADUATE-LEVEL PREPARED HOME HEALTH NURSE AND THE ADVANCED PRACTICE REGISTERED NURSE

The graduate-level prepared home health nurse or the advanced practice registered nurse:

- Integrates innovative and therapeutic interventions in the plan that reflect current evidence, including research, literature, and expert clinical knowledge.

- Provides expert practice, education, and consultation on developing care plans that meet the multifaceted needs of patients with complex problems.

- Leads the design and development of interprofessional practices to address the identified diagnoses, needs, or issues.

- Actively participates in the development and continuous improvement of systems that support the planning process.

Standard 5. Implementation

The home health registered nurse implements the individualized patient plan of care.

COMPETENCIES

The home health registered nurse:

- Collaborates with the patient, family, other caregivers, and interprofessional healthcare team members to implement and integrate the plan in a safe, realistic, and timely manner.

- Assumes responsibility for the safe and efficient implementation of the plan.

- Provides oversight in the implementation of the plan of care.

- Employs strategies to optimize patient engagement and self-management of disease.

- Demonstrates caring behaviors toward patients, family, and caregivers.

- Uses technology to measure, record, and retrieve patient data; implement the nursing process; and enhance nursing practice.

- Uses evidence-based interventions, best practices, and treatments specific to the diagnosis or problem.

- Provides holistic care that addresses the needs of diverse populations across the lifespan and in all settings and transitions.

- Advocates for health care that is sensitive to the needs of patients, families, and caregivers, with particular emphasis on the needs of diverse populations.

- Applies appropriate knowledge and best practices of major health problems and cultural diversity in implementing the plan of care.

- Applies healthcare technologies to maximize access and optimize outcomes for patients and populations.

- Uses community resources and systems to implement and complement the plan of care.

- Accommodates different styles of communication used by patients, families, caregivers, and healthcare team members.

- Integrates traditional and complementary healthcare practices as appropriate.

- Implements the plan in a timely manner, and in accordance with governmental and organizational rules and regulations, to ensure patient safety goals.

- Promotes patient, family, and other caregiver engagement to optimize participation and problem-solving.

- Documents implementation and any modifications to the collaborative plan of care.

ADDITIONAL COMPETENCIES FOR THE GRADUATE-LEVEL PREPARED HOME HEALTH NURSE AND THE ADVANCED PRACTICE REGISTERED NURSE

The graduate-level prepared home health nurse or the advanced practice registered nurse:

- Facilitates utilization of systems, organizations, and community resources to implement the plan.

- Initiates changes in nursing care practices using new knowledge and evidence-based strategies to achieve desired outcomes.

- Acts as a role model to promote therapeutic relationships between healthcare team members and patients, families, and caregivers.

- Actively participates in the development and continuous improvement of systems that support implementation of the plan.

- Uses advanced communication skills to promote relationships among nurses, patients, and patients' families to provide the context for open discussion of the patient's experiences and to improve patient outcomes.

Standard 5A. Coordination of Care

The home health registered nurse coordinates care delivery.

COMPETENCIES

The home health registered nurse:

- Organizes the components of the plan of care.

- Collaborates with other healthcare team members to ensure timely, safe, and efficient implementation and revision of the plan of care.

- Manages a patient's care so as to maximize patient engagement, independence, quality of life, and optimal health.

- Assists the patient, family, and other caregivers to identify options for alternative care when the current plan of care fails to meet the patient's needs or desires.

- Communicates with the patient, family, other caregivers, and other healthcare providers during transitions in care.

- Advocates for the delivery of dignified and humane care by the interprofessional team.

- Documents the coordination of care.

ADDITIONAL COMPETENCIES FOR THE GRADUATE-LEVEL PREPARED HOME HEALTH NURSE AND THE ADVANCED PRACTICE REGISTERED NURSE

The graduate-level prepared home health nurse or the advanced practice registered nurse:

- Provides leadership in the coordination of interprofessional health care for integrated delivery of patient care services.

- Synthesizes data and information to prescribe necessary system and community support measures.

Standard 5B. Health Teaching and Health Promotion

The home health registered nurse employs strategies to promote health and a safe environment.

COMPETENCIES

The home health registered nurse:

- Provides health teaching that addresses such topics as disease management, medication management, healthy lifestyles, risk-reducing behaviors, developmental stages, activities of daily living, immunizations, and health screenings.

- Uses health promotion and health teaching methods appropriate to the situation and the patient's, family's, and caregivers' values, beliefs, health practices, developmental level, learning needs, readiness and ability to learn, language preference, spiritual preferences, culture, and socioeconomic status.

- Encourages patient engagement, especially in self-care management decisions and activities.

- Seeks opportunities for feedback and evaluation of the effectiveness of the strategies used.

- Uses information technologies to communicate health promotion and disease prevention information to the patient in a variety of settings.

- Provides patients with information about intended effects and potential adverse effects of proposed therapies.

ADDITIONAL COMPETENCIES FOR THE GRADUATE-LEVEL PREPARED HOME HEALTH NURSE AND THE ADVANCED PRACTICE REGISTERED NURSE

The graduate-level prepared home health nurse or the advanced practice registered nurse:

- Synthesizes empirical evidence on risk behaviors, learning theories, behavioral change theories, motivational theories, epidemiology, and other related theories and frameworks when designing health education information and programs.

- Conducts personalized health teaching and counseling that considers comparative effectiveness research recommendations.

- Designs health information and patient education appropriate to the patient's developmental level, learning needs, readiness to learn, and cultural values and beliefs.

- Evaluates health information resources for accuracy, readability, and comprehensibility to help patients access quality health information.

- Engages patient alliances and advocacy groups in health teaching and health promotion activities.

- Provides anticipatory guidance and other programs to patients, families, caregivers, and community groups to promote health and prevent or reduce the risk of health problems.

Standard 5C. Consultation

The advanced practice registered nurse provides consultation to influence the identified plan, enhance the abilities of both healthcare providers and the patient, and effect change.

COMPETENCIES FOR THE GRADUATE-LEVEL PREPARED HOME HEALTH NURSE AND THE ADVANCED PRACTICE REGISTERED NURSE

The graduate-level prepared home health nurse or the advanced practice registered nurse:

- Synthesizes clinical data, theoretical frameworks, and evidence when providing consultation.

- Facilitates the effectiveness of a consultation by involving patients, families, and caregivers in decision-making and negotiation of role responsibilities.

- Communicates consultation recommendations effectively.

- Provides education for the healthcare team focusing on high risk, high-tech care, and other complex disease processes and interventions.

Standard 5D. Prescriptive Authority and Treatment

The advanced practice registered nurse uses prescriptive authority, procedures, referrals, treatments, and therapies in accordance with state and federal laws and regulations.

ADDITIONAL COMPETENCIES FOR THE GRADUATE-LEVEL PREPARED HOME HEALTH NURSE AND THE ADVANCED PRACTICE REGISTERED NURSE

The graduate-level prepared home health nurse or the advanced practice registered nurse:

- Prescribes evidence-based treatments, therapies, and procedures considering the patient's comprehensive healthcare needs.

- Prescribes pharmacologic agents according to a current knowledge of pharmacology and physiology.

- Prescribes specific pharmacologic agents or treatments based on clinical indicators, the patient's status and needs, and the results of diagnostic and laboratory tests.

- Evaluates therapeutic and potential adverse effects of pharmacologic and nonpharmacologic treatments.

- Provides patients, families, and caregivers with information about intended effects and potential adverse effects of proposed prescriptive therapies.

- Provides information about costs and alternative treatments and procedures, as appropriate.

- Evaluates and incorporates complementary and alternative therapy into education and practice.

Standard 6. Evaluation

The home health registered nurse evaluates progress toward attainment of outcomes.

COMPETENCIES

The home health registered nurse:

- Conducts a systematic, ongoing, and criterion-based evaluation of the outcomes in relation to the structures and processes prescribed by the plan of care and the indicated timeline.

- Engages the patient and others involved in the care or situation in the evaluation process.

- Evaluates, in partnership with the patient, the effectiveness of the planned strategies in relation to the patient's responses and attainment of the expected outcomes.

- Evaluates the patient's achievement of short-term goals that empower self-efficacy.

- Uses ongoing assessment data to revise the diagnoses, outcomes, plan, and implementation strategies.

- Disseminates evaluation results to the patient, family, other caregivers, and other healthcare providers involved, in accordance with federal and state regulations.

- Promotes use of appropriate interventions to minimize patient suffering and avoid unwanted treatment.

- Documents the results of the evaluation.

ADDITIONAL COMPETENCIES FOR THE GRADUATE-LEVEL PREPARED HOME HEALTH NURSE AND THE ADVANCED PRACTICE REGISTERED NURSE

The graduate-level prepared home health nurse or the advanced practice registered nurse:

- Evaluates the accuracy of the diagnosis and the effectiveness of the interventions and other variables in relation to the patient's attainment of expected outcomes.

- Synthesizes the results of evaluations to determine the effect of the plan on patients, families, groups, communities, and institutions.

- Adapts the plan of care for the trajectory of treatment according to evaluation of the response.

- Uses the results of the evaluation to make or recommend process or structural changes, including policy, procedure, or protocol revision, as appropriate.

Standards of Professional Performance for Home Health Nursing

Standard 7. Ethics

The home health registered nurse practices ethically.

COMPETENCIES
The home health registered nurse:

- Uses *Code of Ethics for Nurses with Interpretive Statements* (ANA, 2001) to guide practice.

- Delivers care in a manner that preserves and protects patient autonomy, dignity, rights, values, and beliefs.

- Recognizes the centrality of the patient and family as core members of any healthcare team.

- Upholds patient confidentiality within legal and regulatory parameters.

- Assists patients in self-determination and informed decision-making.

- Provides information on the patient's rights and responsibilities, as well as risks, benefits, and outcomes of healthcare regimens, to allow informed decision-making by the patient, including informed consent and informed refusal.

- Maintains a therapeutic and professional patient–nurse relationship within appropriate professional role boundaries.

- Contributes to resolving ethical issues involving patients, colleagues, community groups, systems, and other stakeholders.

- Takes appropriate action regarding instances of illegal, unethical, or inappropriate behavior that could endanger or jeopardize the best interests of patients or situations.

- Speaks up to question healthcare practice when necessary for safety and quality improvement.

- Advocates for equitable patient care.
- Maintains her or his own health and well-being through health-promoting behaviors.

ADDITIONAL COMPETENCIES FOR THE GRADUATE-LEVEL PREPARED HOME HEALTH NURSE AND THE ADVANCED PRACTICE REGISTERED NURSE

The graduate-level prepared home health nurse or the advanced practice registered nurse:

- Participates in interprofessional teams that address ethical risks, benefits, and outcomes.
- Promotes excellence in clinical practice that supports accuracy and truthfulness in coding, financing, and reporting of outcomes at the agency and systems level.
- Uses expertise to influence health policy.

Standard 8. Education

The home health registered nurse attains knowledge and competence that reflect current nursing practice.

COMPETENCIES
The home health registered nurse:

- Participates in ongoing educational activities to keep abreast of professional practice issues, knowledge, and skills to provide evidence-based patient care.

- Demonstrates a commitment to lifelong learning through self-reflective inquiry that addresses personal learning and professional growth needs.

- Seeks relevant educational experiences that reflect current practice needs to maintain current knowledge, skills, abilities, and judgment in clinical practice or role performance.

- Acquires evidence-based knowledge and skills appropriate to the population, specialty, setting, role, or situation.

- Seeks formal and independent learning experiences to develop and maintain current knowledge, clinical skills, and professional skills.

- Identifies learning needs based on nursing knowledge, the various roles the nurse may assume, and the changing needs of the population.

- Participates in formal or informal consultations to address issues in nursing practice as an application of education and knowledge base.

- Shares educational findings, experiences, and ideas with peers.

- Contributes to a work environment conducive to the education of healthcare professionals.

- Maintains professional records that provide evidence of competence and lifelong learning.

ADDITIONAL COMPETENCIES FOR THE GRADUATE-LEVEL PREPARED HOME HEALTH NURSE AND THE ADVANCED PRACTICE REGISTERED NURSE

The graduate-level prepared home health nurse or the advanced practice registered nurse:

- Uses current healthcare research findings and other evidence to expand clinical knowledge, skills, abilities, and judgment; enhance role performance; contribute to innovative practice models and improved patient outcomes; and increase knowledge of professional issues.

- Provides education and consultation to other home health clinicians regarding strategies to enhance patient care and improve the disease self-management skills of patients, families, and caregivers.

Standard 9. Evidence-Based Practice and Research

The home health registered nurse integrates evidence and research findings into practice.

COMPETENCIES

The home health registered nurse:

- Uses current evidence-based nursing knowledge, including research findings, to guide practice.

- Incorporates evidence when initiating changes in nursing practice.

- Participates, as appropriate to educational level and position, in the formulation of evidence-based practice through research.

- Shares personal or third-party research findings with colleagues and peers.

ADDITIONAL COMPETENCIES FOR THE GRADUATE-LEVEL PREPARED HOME HEALTH NURSE AND THE ADVANCED PRACTICE REGISTERED NURSE

The graduate-level prepared home health nurse or the advanced practice registered nurse:

- Contributes to nursing knowledge by conducting or synthesizing research and other evidence that discovers, examines, and evaluates current practice, knowledge, theories, criteria, and creative approaches to improve healthcare outcomes.

- Promotes a climate of research and clinical inquiry within the interprofessional healthcare team and the community.

- Disseminates research findings through activities such as presentations, publications, consultation, and journal clubs.

Standard 10. Quality of Practice

The home health registered nurse contributes to quality nursing practice.

COMPETENCIES

The home health registered nurse:

- Demonstrates quality by applying and documenting the nursing process in a responsible, accountable, and ethical manner.

- Uses best practices, creativity, and innovation to enhance the quality of care and improve patient outcomes.

- Participates in quality improvement initiatives in home health nursing and interprofessional practice. Activities may include:

  - Identifying aspects of practice important for quality monitoring.

  - Using indicators to monitor quality, safety, and effectiveness of practice.

  - Collecting data to monitor quality and effectiveness of practice.

  - Analyzing quality data to identify opportunities for improving practice.

  - Formulating recommendations to improve practice and outcomes.

  - Implementing activities to enhance the quality of practice.

  - Developing, implementing, and/or evaluating policies, procedures, and guidelines to improve the quality of practice.

  - Leading interprofessional teams to evaluate clinical care and health services.

  - Participating in efforts to minimize costs and support appropriate resource utilization.

  - Identifying problems that occur in day-to-day work routines in order to correct process inefficiencies.*

* Board of Higher Education & Massachusetts Organization of Nurse Executives (BHE/MONE), 2006.

- Analyzing factors related to quality, safety, and effectiveness.
- Analyzing organizational systems for barriers to quality patient outcomes.
- Implementing processes to remove or weaken barriers within organizational systems.

ADDITIONAL COMPETENCIES FOR THE GRADUATE-LEVEL PREPARED HOME HEALTH NURSE AND THE ADVANCED PRACTICE REGISTERED NURSE

The graduate-level prepared home health nurse or the advanced practice registered nurse:

- Provides leadership in the design and implementation of quality improvements.
- Designs innovations to effect change in practice and improve health outcomes.
- Evaluates the practice environment and quality of nursing care rendered in relation to existing evidence and best practices.
- Identifies opportunities for the generation and use of research and evidence.
- Obtains and maintains relevant professional certification(s).
- Uses the results of quality improvement activities to initiate changes in home health nursing practice and the healthcare delivery system.

Standard 11. Communication

The home health registered nurse communicates effectively in a variety of formats in all areas of practice.

COMPETENCIES

The home health registered nurse:

- Assesses communication format preferences of patients, families, and colleagues.*

- Assesses the language and literacy needs of patients, families, and caregivers, such as the need to use interpreters, translated education resources, and low-literacy patient education materials.

- Assesses her or his own communication skills in encounters with patients, families, caregivers, and colleagues.

- Seeks continuous improvement of her or his own communication and conflict resolution skills.*

- Develops communication skills that promote behavior change in patients, such as the use of motivational interviewing, counseling, and health coaching communication techniques.

- Conveys information to patients, families, caregivers, the interprofessional team, and others in communication formats that promote accuracy and accommodate patient privacy.

- Questions the rationale supporting care processes and decisions when they do not appear to be in the best interest of the patient.*

- Discloses observations or concerns related to hazards and errors in care or the practice environment to the appropriate level.

- Assesses the urgency of communicating information to patients, family, caregivers, and other healthcare team members.

- Maintains communication with other interprofessional healthcare team members to minimize risks associated with transfers and transition in care delivery.

- Contributes her or his own professional perspective in discussions with the interprofessional team.

* BHE/MONE, 2006.

Standard 12. Leadership

The home health registered nurse demonstrates leadership in the professional practice setting and the profession.

COMPETENCIES

The home health registered nurse:

- Treats patients, family members, and caregivers respectfully and courteously, while supporting their engagement in self-care and caregiving skills.

- Treats colleagues with respect, trust, and dignity.

- Trusts colleagues to be accountable for the care and services they provide.

- Develops communication and conflict resolution skills.

- Communicates effectively with patients, family members, caregivers, and colleagues by proactively addressing issues and by using conflict management skills to courteously resolve differences.

- Abides by the vision, the associated goals, and the plan to implement and measure progress of the patient within the context of the home health agency and healthcare organization.

- Coordinates the nursing care given by others while addressing the quality of that care.

- Incorporates the home health agency's quality initiatives into patients' goals and care planning, and measures patients' progress in meeting those quality goals.

- Inspires quality care while coordinating patient care given by caregivers, paraprofessionals, and other team members.

- Precepts colleagues, including those new to home health practice, for the advancement of home health nursing practice, the profession, and quality health care.

- Participates in the education of nursing students and serves as a role model.

- Participates in the home health agency's committees and quality teams to enhance home health policies, standards, and practices.

- Promotes the mission and vision of the health agency among colleagues.

- Demonstrates a commitment to continuous lifelong learning and education for self and others.

- Seeks ways to advance nursing autonomy and accountability.*

- Participates in efforts to influence healthcare policy involving patients and the profession.

- Participates in professional nursing and home health organizations to influence healthcare policy and advance the profession and the care of patients in their homes.

- Models collegial behaviors, including trust, courtesy, and respectful communications.

ADDITIONAL COMPETENCIES FOR THE GRADUATE-LEVEL PREPARED HOME HEALTH NURSE AND THE ADVANCED PRACTICE REGISTERED NURSE

The graduate-level prepared home health nurse or the advanced practice registered nurse:

- Models expert practice to interprofessional team members and healthcare consumers.

- Provides direction to enhance the effectiveness of the interprofessional team.

- Initiates discussions within the home health agency about ways to enhance the professional practice environment and patient outcomes.

- Contributes to decision-making within the agency and with system-wide and community organizations to advance policies and practices that enhance patient outcomes.

- Mentors colleagues in the acquisition of clinical knowledge, skills, abilities, and judgment.

- Promotes advanced practice nursing and role development by interpreting its role for patients, families, caregivers, colleagues, and policy-makers.

- Influences decision-making within the organization to improve the professional practice environment and patient outcomes.

* BHE/MONE, 2006.

Standard 13. Collaboration

The home health registered nurse collaborates with patients, families, caregivers, interprofessional healthcare teams, and others in the conduct of nursing practice.

COMPETENCIES
The home health registered nurse:

- Partners with others to effect change and produce positive outcomes through the sharing of knowledge of the patient and/or situation.

- Communicates with the patient, family, other caregivers, and healthcare team members regarding home health care and the home health nurse's role in the provision of that care.

- Engages the patient, family, and other caregivers in attaining self-care management, knowledge, skills, and responsibility for outcomes.

- Participates in coordination of care, building consensus or resolving conflict in the context of patient care.

- Applies group process and negotiation techniques with patients, families, caregivers, and the interprofessional healthcare team to achieve outcomes.

- Adheres to standards and applicable codes of conduct that govern behavior among healthcare team members, peers, and colleagues to create a work environment that promotes cooperation, respect, and trust.

- Leads communication and cooperative efforts in creating an interprofessional plan of care focused on outcomes, while engaging patients, families, caregivers, and others in the care and delivery of services.

- Engages in teamwork and team-building processes.

ADDITIONAL COMPETENCIES FOR THE GRADUATE-LEVEL PREPARED HOME HEALTH NURSE AND THE ADVANCED PRACTICE REGISTERED NURSE
The graduate-level prepared home health nurse or the advanced practice registered nurse:

- Partners with other members of the healthcare system to enhance patient outcomes through interprofessional activities, such as education, consultation, management, technological development, or research opportunities.

- Invites the contribution of the patient, family, other caregivers, and team members to agency and system-wide initiatives to achieve optimal outcomes.

- Leads in establishing, improving, and sustaining collaborative relationships throughout the healthcare system to achieve safe, quality care.

- Documents plan-of-care communications, rationales for plan-of-care changes, and collaborative discussions to improve patient outcomes.

Standard 14. Professional Practice Evaluation

The home health registered nurse evaluates one's own nursing practice in relation to professional practice standards and guidelines, relevant statutes, rules, and regulations.

COMPETENCIES
The home health registered nurse:

- Provides age-appropriate and developmentally appropriate care in a culturally and ethnically sensitive manner.

- Engages in self-evaluation of practice on a regular basis, identifying areas of strength as well as areas in which professional growth would be beneficial.

- Obtains informal feedback regarding her or his own practice from patients, families, caregivers, peers, professional colleagues, and others.

- Participates in peer review activities, such as chart review.

- Takes action to achieve goals identified during the evaluation process.

- Provides rationale and evidence for practice decisions and actions as part of the informal and formal evaluation processes.

- Interacts with peers and colleagues to enhance her or his own professional nursing practice or role performance.

- Provides peers with formal or informal constructive feedback regarding their practice or role performance.

ADDITIONAL COMPETENCIES FOR THE GRADUATE-LEVEL PREPARED HOME HEALTH NURSE AND THE ADVANCED PRACTICE REGISTERED NURSE
The graduate-level prepared home health nurse or the advanced practice registered nurse:

- Engages in a formal process seeking feedback regarding her or his own practice from patients, families, caregivers, peers, professional colleagues, and others.

Standard 15. Resource Utilization

The home health registered nurse uses appropriate resources to plan and provide nursing services that are safe, effective, and financially responsible.

COMPETENCIES

The home health registered nurse:

- Assesses patient, family, and other caregiver needs and resources available to implement the plan of care and to achieve desired outcomes.

- Identifies patient, family, and other caregiver abilities and competencies, including potential for harm, complexity of the task, and desired outcome, when considering resource allocation.

- Delegates elements of care to appropriate clinical team members to achieve excellent care at the least cost in accordance with any applicable legal or policy parameters or principles.

- Identifies the evidence when evaluating resources.

- Evaluates the evidence of resource effectiveness and cost when developing the plan of care.

- Advocates for resources, including technology, that enhance home health nursing practice.

- Modifies practice to promote positive interaction among patient, family, caregivers, and technology.

- Assists the patient and family in identifying and securing appropriate services to address needs across the healthcare continuum.

- Assists the patient and family in factoring costs, risks, and benefits in decisions about treatment and care at home.

ADDITIONAL COMPETENCIES FOR THE GRADUATE-LEVEL PREPARED HOME HEALTH NURSE AND THE ADVANCED PRACTICE REGISTERED NURSE

The graduate-level prepared home health nurse or the advanced practice registered nurse:

- Uses organizational and community resources to formulate interprofessional plans of care that support appropriate utilization of services.

- Formulates innovative solutions for patient care problems that use agency and community resources effectively while promoting quality care.

- Designs evaluation strategies that demonstrate cost effectiveness, cost benefit, and efficiency factors associated with nursing, the clinical team, and community resources.

- Develops programs in collaboration with other community-based organizations to meet the needs of patients, families, and caregivers that enhance achievement of patient outcomes while accessing home health and other services across the continuum of care.

Standard 16. Environmental Health

The home health registered nurse practices in an environmentally safe and healthy manner.

COMPETENCIES

The home health registered nurse:

- Attains knowledge of how environmental health concepts and strategies are applied in the home health care practice setting, especially as related to needles, syringes, drugs, medications, and waste management.

- Advocates for the judicious and appropriate use and disposal of products used in patient care.

- Assesses the patient's home and community for safety and risk factors, such as unsafe homes and neighborhoods, unsanitary conditions, and animals and pests that threaten the health of patients, families, caregivers, or home health agency staff.

- Promotes a practice environment that reduces environmental health risks for patients, caregivers, home health team members, and the community.

- Communicates environmental health risks and exposure reduction strategies to patients, families, caregivers, colleagues, and communities.

- Utilizes scientific evidence to determine if a product or treatment is an environmental threat.

- Participates in strategies to promote healthy communities.

ADDITIONAL COMPETENCIES FOR THE GRADUATE-LEVEL PREPARED HOME HEALTH NURSE AND THE ADVANCED PRACTICE REGISTERED NURSE

The graduate-level prepared home health nurse or the advanced practice registered nurse:

- Initiates practices within the home and home health organization that prevent risk and injury of patients, caregivers, and the community, such as implementation of safe patient handling and mobility principles.

- Identifies areas of policy or practice that jeopardize the health of the healthcare team, patients, families, caregivers, or the community within the environment.

- Designs policies and procedures that promote best practices in creating a safe environment for patients, caregivers, and communities.

- Analyzes the impact of social, political, and economic influences on the environment and human health exposures.

- Promotes long-term solutions when addressing issues related to environmental health and the environment in which patients, home health staff, and their communities live and work.

- Creates partnerships that promote sustainable environmental health policies and conditions.

- Critically evaluates the manner in which environmental health issues are presented by the popular media.

- Advocates for implementation of environmental principles for nursing practice.

- Supports nurses in advocating for and implementing environmental principles in nursing practice.

Glossary

Care coordination. The deliberate organization of patient care activities between two or more participants (including the patient) involved in the patient's care to facilitate the appropriate delivery of health services. This involves the marshalling of personnel and other resources needed to carry out all required patient care activities and is often managed by the exchange of information among participants responsible for different aspects of care. (McDonald, et al., 2010; pg. 4.)

Care/management. The application of systems, science, incentives, and information to improve medical practice and assist healthcare consumers and their support system to become engaged in a collaborative process to manage medical, social, and mental health conditions more effectively. Its goal is to achieve an optimal level of wellness and improve coordination of care while providing cost-effective, non-duplicative services. (Adapted from WHCA, 2008.)

Caregivers. Those persons, including family members, friends, neighbors, or privately paid individuals, who provide assistance to patients.

Continuity of care. An interprofessional communication process that promotes patient safety and well-being across settings and transitions of care. This process includes patients, families, and caregivers in the development of a coordinated plan of care.

Evidence-based practice. Applying the best available synthesis of research results (evidence) in healthcare decision-making. Healthcare professionals who perform EBP use research evidence along with clinical expertise and patient preferences. Systematic reviews (summaries of healthcare research results) further informs the EBP process. (Adapted from AHRQ, n.d.)

Family. The family of origin or designated others as identified by the patient.

Interprofessional. A collaborative approach that relies on the overlapping knowledge, skills, and abilities of each professional team member. This synergistic and comprehensive approach can enhance outcomes that exceed the individual efforts of the team members.

Meaningful use. The set of standards defined by the Centers for Medicare & Medicaid Services (CMS) Incentive Programs that governs the use of electronic health records and allows eligible providers and hospitals to earn incentive payments by meeting specific criteria (CMS, n.d.).

Medical home. Model of care that emphasizes care coordination and communication to transform primary care into "what patients want it to be" (NCQA, n.d.)

Nurse coach. A registered nurse who integrates coaching competencies into any setting or specialty area of practice to facilitate a process of change or development that assists individuals or groups to realize their potential (Hess et al., 2013, p. 52).

Nurse coaching. A skilled, purposeful, results-oriented, and structured relationship-centered interaction with clients provided by registered nurses for the purpose of promoting achievement of client goals (Hess et al., 2013, p. 52).

Patient engagement. "'[A]ctions individuals must take to obtain the greatest benefit from the health care services available to them.' This definition focuses on behaviors of individuals relative to their health care that are critical and proximal to health outcomes, rather than the actions of professionals or policies of institutions" (Center for Advancing Health, 2010).

References

Agency for Healthcare Research and Quality (AHRQ, n.d.) *Glossary of Terms*. Retrieved from http://effectivehealthcare.ahrq.gov/index.cfm/glossary-of-terms/?pageaction=showterm&termid=24

American Nurses Association. (1986). *Standards of home health nursing*. Kansas City, MO: American Nurses Association.

American Nurses Association. (1992). *Scope of practice for home health nursing*. Kansas City, MO: American Nurses Association.

American Nurses Association. (1999). *Scope and standards of home health nursing practice*. Washington, DC: American Nurses Association.

American Nurses Association. (2001). *Code of ethics for nurses with interpretive statements*. Washington, DC: Nursesbooks.org.

American Nurses Association. (2008). *Home health nursing: Scope and standards of practice*. Silver Spring, MD: Nursesbooks.org.

American Nurses Association. (2010a). *Nursing: Scope and standards of practice, second edition*. Silver Spring, MD: Nursesbooks.org.

American Nurses Association. (2010b). *Nursing's social policy statement: The essence of the profession*. Silver Spring, MD: Nursesbooks.org.

American Nurses Association. (2013a). *ANA recognized terminologies that support nursing practice*. Retrieved from http://www.nursingworld.org/terminologies

American Nurses Association. (2013b). *Safe patient handling and mobility: Interprofessional national standards across the care continuum*. Silver Spring, MD: Nursesbooks.org.

American Nurses Credentialing Center (ANCC). (n.d.). Magnet recognition program model. Retrieved from http://www.nursecredentialing.org/Magnet/ProgramOverview/New-Magnet-Model

REFERENCES

American Nurses Credentialing Center (ANCC). (n.d.). Pathway to excellence: Practice standards. Retrieved from http://www.nursecredentialing.org/Pathway/AboutPathway/PathwayPracticeStandards

Association for Professionals in Infection Control and Epidemiology (APIC) Home Care Membership Section, Embry, F. C., Chinnes, L. F., et al. (2008). *APIC-HICPAC surveillance definitions for home health care and home hospice infections.* Retrieved from http://www.apic.org/resource_/tinymcefilemanager/practice_guidance/hh-surv-def.pdf

Auer, P., & Nirenberg, A. (2008). Nurse practitioner home-based primary care: A model for the care of frail elders. *Clinical Scholars Review, 1*(1), 33–39.

Bergquist-Beringer, S., & Gajewski, B. J. (2011) Outcome and Assessment Information Set data that predict pressure ulcer development in older adult home health patients. *Advances in Skin and Wound Care, 24*(9), 404–414.

Berwick, D. M., Nolan, T. W., & Whittington, J. (2008). The Triple Aim: Care, health, and cost. *Health Affairs, 27*(3), 759–769.

Blumenthal, D., & Tavenner, M. (2010). The "meaningful use" regulation for electronic health records. *New England Journal of Medicine, 363*(6), 501–504.

Board of Higher Education & Massachusetts Organization of Nurse Executives (BHE/MONE). (2006). *Creativity and connections: Building the framework for the future of nursing education.* Report from the Invitational Working Session, March 23–24, 2006. Burlington, MA: MONE. Retrieved from http://www.mass.edu/currentinit/documents/NursingCreativityAndConnections.pdf

Bowles, K. H., Potashnik, S., Ratchliff, S. J., Rosenberg, M., Shih, N.-W., Topaz, M., . . . , Naylor, M. D. (2013). Conducting research using the electronic health record across multi-hospital systems. *Journal of Nursing Administration, 43*(6), 355–360.

Briggs Corporation. (2006). Briggs® national quality improvement/hospitalization reduction study. Retrieved from http://www.briggscorp.com/ACHstrategies/BriggsStudy.pdf

Buhler-Wilkerson, K. (2003). *No place like home. A history of nursing and home care in the United States.* Baltimore, MD: Johns Hopkins University Press.

REFERENCES

Buhler-Wilkerson, K. (2012). No place like home. A history of nursing and home care in the United States. *Home Healthcare Nurse, 30*(8), 446–452.

Bureau of Labor Statistics. (2010). Occupational outlook handbook: Registered nurses. Retrieved from http://www.bls.gov/ooh/healthcare/registered-nurses.htm#tab-3

Calys, M., Gagnon, K., & Jernigan, S. (2012), A validation study of the Missouri Alliance for Home Care fall risk assessment tool. *Home Health Care Management & Practice, 25*(2), 39–44.

Candy, B., Holman, A., Leurent, B., Davis, S., & Jones, L. (2011). Hospice care delivered at home, in nursing homes and in dedicated hospice facilities: A systematic review of quantitative and qualitative evidence. *International Journal of Nursing Studies, 48*(1), 121–133.

Center for Advancing Health. (2010). *A new definition of patient engagement: What is engagement and why is it important?* Retrieved from http://www.cfah.org/pdfs/CFAH_Engagement_Behavior_Framework_current.pdf

Centers for Disease Control and Prevention (CDC). (2012). Use and characteristics of electronic health records systems among office-based physician practices: United States, 2001–2012. Retrieved from http://www.cdc.gov/nchs/data/databriefs/db111.htm

Centers for Medicare & Medicaid Services (CMS). (n.d.). Retrieved from http://www.healthit.gov/policy-researchers-implementers/meaningful-use

Commission on Chronic Illness. (1956–1959). *Chronic illness in the United States* (4 vols.). Cambridge, MA: Harvard University Press.

Corbett, C. F., Setter, S. M., Daratha, K. B., Nuemiller, J. J., & Wood, L. D. (2010). Nurse-identified hospital to home medication discrepancies: Implications for improving transitional care. *Geriatric Nursing, 31*(3), 188–196.

Craven, Mrs. Dacre [Florence Sarah Lees]. (1889). *A guide to district nurses and home visiting.* London & New York: Macmillan.

Dieckmann, J. L. (2012). History of public health and public and community health nursing. In M. Stanhope & J. Lancaster (Eds.), *Public health nursing: Population-centered health care in the community* (8th ed., pp. 22–43). Maryland Heights, MO: Mosby-Elsevier.

REFERENCES

Doran, G. T. (1981). There's a S.M.A.R.T. way to write management's goals and objectives. *Management Review, 70*(11), 35–36.

Dwyer, L. L., Harris-Kojetin, L. D., Valverde, R. H., Frazier, J. M., Simon, A. E., Stone, N. D., & Thompson, N. D. (2013). Infections in long-term care populations in the United States. *Journal of the American Geriatrics Society, 61*(3), 341–349.

Fazzi Associates. (2009, October). The Blackberry report: The national state of the home care industry. Retrieved from http://www.leadinghomecare.com/blog.2009/10/blackberry-report-national-state-of.html

Fazzi Associates. (2013). National state of the industry: Home care and hospice. Retrieved from http://www.fazzi.com/id-2013-state-of-the-home-care-industry-study.html

Friedman, D. J., Parrish, R. G., & Ross, D. A. (2013). Electronic health records and US public health: Current realities and future promise. *American Journal of Public Health, 103*(9), 1560–1567.

Gomes, B., Calanzani, N., Curiale, V., McCrone, P., & Higginson, I. J. (2013, June 6). Effectiveness and cost-effectiveness of home-based palliative care services for adults with advanced illness and their caregivers. *Cochrane Database of Systematic Reviews, 6*, Art. No. CD007760.

Hall, P. B., Poole, R., & Hall, C. A. (2013, September). Bridging the gaps in supportive information systems. *Home Healthcare Nurse, 31*(8), 419–428.

Harris, M. (Ed). (2001). *Home Healthcare Nurses' Association's Core Curriculum*. Washington, DC: National Association for Home Care.

Harris, M. (2010). *Handbook of home health care administration, fifth edition*. Sudbury, MA: Jones & Bartlett.

Harris, M. (2013, April). We need your input . . . this is your opportunity to have a voice in the future of your profession [Guest editorial]. *Home Healthcare Nurse, 31*(4), 177–180.

Heeke, S., Wood, F., & Schuck, J. (2014). Improving care transitions from hospital to home: Standardized orders for home health nursing with remote telemonitoring. *Journal of Nursing Care Quality 29*(2), E21–28.

Hess, D. R, Dossey, B. M., et al. (2013). *The art and science of nurse coaching: The provider's guide to coaching scope and competencies*. Silver Spring, MD: Nursesbooks.org.

Hoban, M. B., Fedor, M., Reeder, S., & Chernick, M. (2013, July/August). The effect of telemonitoring at home on quality of life and self-care behaviors of patients with heart failure. *Home Healthcare Nurse, 31*(7), 368–377.

Institute of Medicine (IOM). (2010). *The future of nursing: Leading change, advancing health.* Washington, DC: National Academy of Sciences.

Madigan, E. A., Gordon, N. H., Fortinsky, R. H., Koroukian, S. M., Piña, I., & Riggs, J. S. (2012). Rehospitalization in a national population of home health care patients with heart failure. *Health Services Research, 47*(6), 2316–2338.

Madigan, E. A., Schmotzer, B. J., Struk, C. J., DiCarlo, C. M., Kikano, G., Pina, I. L., & Boxer, R. S. (2013). Home health care with telemonitoring improves health status for older adults with heart failure. *Home Health Care Services Quarterly, 32*(1), 57–74.

Madigan, E. A., & Vanderboom, C. (2005). Home health nursing research priorities. *Applied Nursing Research, 18*(4), 221–225.

Martin, K. S. (2005). *The Omaha System: A key to practice, documentation, and information management* (reprinted 2nd ed.). Omaha, NE: Health Connections Press.

Martin, K. S., & Utterback, K. B. (2014). Home health and related community-based systems. In R. Nelson & N. Staggers, *Health informatics: An interprofessional approach* (pp. 147–163). St. Louis, MO: Elsevier.

Masotti, P., McColl, M. A., & Green, M. (2010). Adverse events experienced by homecare patients: A scoping review of the literature. *International Journal for Quality in Health Care, 22*(10), 115–125.

McClelland, M., McCoy, M., & Burson, R. (2013). Clinical nurse specialists: Then, now, and the future of the profession. *Clinical Nurse Specialist, 27*(2), 96–102.

McDonald, K. M., Schultz, E., Albin, L., Pineda N., Lonhart J., Sundaram V., Smith-Spangler C., Brustrom J., & Malcolm, E. *Care coordination atlas. Version 3.* (2010) (Prepared by Stanford University subcontract to Battelle on Contract No. 290-04-0020). AHRQ Publication No. 11-0023-EF. Rockville, MD: Agency for Healthcare Research and Quality. November 2010. Retrieved from http://www.ahrq.gov/professionals/systems/long-term-care/resources/coordination/atlas/care-coordination-measures-atlas.pdf

REFERENCES

Medical News Today. (2012). Electronic health record use in US hospitals has doubled in last two years. Retrieved from http://www.medicalnewstoday.com/articles241871.php

Monsen, K. A., & deBlok, J. (2013). Buurtzorg Nederland. *American Journal of Nursing, 113*(8), 55–59.

Monsen, K. A., & Kerr, M. J. (2004). Mining quality documentation for golden outcomes. *Home Health Management and Practice, 16*(3), 192–199.

Monsen, K. A., Westra, B. L., Oancea, S. C., Yu, F., & Kerr, M. J. (2011) Linking home care interventions and hospitalization outcomes for frail and non-frail elderly patients. *Research in Nursing and Health 34*(2), 160–168.

National Association for Home Care & Hospice (NAHC). (2006, January). Briggs national quality improvement/hospitalization reduction study. Retrieved from http://www.nahc.org/NAHC/CaringComm/eNAHCReport/datacharts/hospredstudy.pdf

National Association of Clinical Nurse Specialists (NACNS). (2010). *Clinical nurse specialist core competencies.* Retrieved from http://www.nacns.org/docs/CNSCoreCompetenciesBroch.pdf

National Institute for Healthcare Safety and Health (NIHSH). (2010). *Occupational hazards in home healthcare.* Retrieved from http://www.cdc.gov/niosh/docs/2010-125/pdfs/2010-125.pdf

Naylor, M. D., Bowles, K. H., McCauley, K. M., Maccoy, M. C., Maislin, G., Pauly, M. V., & Krakauer, R. (2011, September). High-value transitional care: Translation of research into practice. *Journal of Evaluation in Clinical Practice, 19*(5), 1–12.

Naylor, M. D., Stephens, C., Bowles, K. H., & Bixby, M. B. (2005). Cognitively impaired older adults: From hospital to home. *American Journal of Nursing, 105*(2), 52–61.

Neal-Boyan, L. (2001, partially revised in 2009). *Core curriculum for home health care nursing.* Washington, DC: Home Healthcare Nurses Association.

Nelson, R., & Staggers, N. (2014). *Health informatics: An interprofessional approach.* St. Louis, MO: Elsevier.

REFERENCES

Nightingale, F. (1859). *Notes on nursing: What it is and what it is not.* London, England. [reprinted by many publishers].

NCQA. (n.d.). [Definition of *medical home*]. Retrieved from http://www.ncqa.org/Programs/Recognition/PatientCenteredMedicalHomePCMH.aspx

O'Connor, M., & Davitt, J. K. (2012). The Outcome and Assessment Information Set (OASIS): A review of validity and reliability. *Home Health Care Services Quarterly, 31*(4), 267–301.

Omaha System. (2013). *References.* Retrieved from http://www.omahasystem.org/references.html

Plemmons, S., Lipton, B., Fong, Y., & Acosta, N. (2012). Measureable outcomes from standardized nursing documentation in an electronic health record. *ANIA-CARING, 27*(2), 4–7.

Registered Nurse Association of Ontario. (2010). Nursing care of dyspnea: The 6th vital sign in individuals with chronic obstructive pulmonary disease. Retrieved from http://rnao.ca/bpg/guidelines/dyspnea

Rogers, E. M. (1995). *Diffusion of innovation* (4th ed.). New York, NY: Free Press.

Schlachta-Fairchild, L., Rocca, M., Cordi, V., Haught, A., Castelli, D., MacMahon, K., . . . , Arnaert, A. (2014). Telehealth and applications for delivering care at a distance. In R. Nelson & N. Staggers, *Health informatics: An interprofessional approach* (pp. 125–146). St. Louis, MO: Elsevier.

Siegel, J. D., Rhinehart, E., Jackson, M., & Chiarello, L. (2007). Guideline for isolation precautions: Preventing transmission of infectious agents in healthcare settings. Retrieved from http://www.cdc.gov/hicpac/pdf/isolation/isolation2007.pdf

Spoelstra, S. L., Given, B., You, M., & Given, C. W. (2012). The contribution falls have to increasing risk of nursing home placement in community dwelling older adults. *Clinical Nursing Research, 21*(1), 24–42.

Suter, P., Gorski, L., Hennessy, B., & Suter, N. (2012). Best practices for heart failure: A focused review. *Home Healthcare Nurse, 30*(7), 394–405.

REFERENCES

Suter, P., & Hennessey, B. (2011). Effective use of technology to engage both patients and provider partners. *CARING, 30*(8), 81–86.

Topaz, M., Golfenshtein, N., & Bowles, K. H. (2014). The Omaha System: A systematic review of the recent literature. *Journal of the American Medical Informatics Association, 21*(1), 163–170.

Transitional Care Model. (n.d.). Retrieved from http://www.nursing.upenn.edu/media/transitionalcare/Documents/Information%20on%20the%20Model.pdf

U.S. Department of Health and Human Services (U.S. DHHS). (2013). *Telehealth*. Retrieved from http://www.hrsa.gov/ruralhealth/about/telehealth/telehealth.html

Vincent, A. E., & Birkhead, A. C. (2013). Evaluation of the effectiveness of nurse coaching in improving health outcomes in chronic conditions. *Holistic Nursing Practice, 27*(3), 148–161.

Visiting Nurse Associations of America (VNAA). (2013). *VNAA blueprint for excellence: Patient engagement.* Retrieved from http://www.vnaablueprint.org/patient-engagement_1.html

Visiting Nurse Service (VNS) of New York. (2013). *VNSNY research*. Retrieved from http://www.vnsny.org/vnsny-research

Washington Health Care Authority (WHCA). (2008). *Operational definition of care management.* Office of Quality and Care Management. Olympia, WA: Author. Retrieved from http://www.hca.wa.gov/medicaid/healthyoptions/documents/ccm_finalopdef.pdf

Westra, B. L., Dey, S., Fang, G., Steinbach, M., Kumar, V., Savik, K., . . . , Dierich, M. (2011, March). Interpretable predictive models for knowledge discovery from home-care electronic health records. *Journal of Healthcare Engineering, 2*(1), 55–74.

White, M., Garbez, R., Carroll, M., Brinker, E., & Howie-Esquivel, J. (2013). Is "teach-back" associated with knowledge retention and hospital readmission in hospitalized heart failure patients? *Journal of Cardiovascular Nursing, 28*(2), 137–146.

Woods, L. W., & Snow, S. W. (2013). The impact of telehealth monitoring. *Home Healthcare Nurse, 31*(1), 39–45.

Appendix A.

Home Health Nursing: Scope and Standards of Practice (2007)

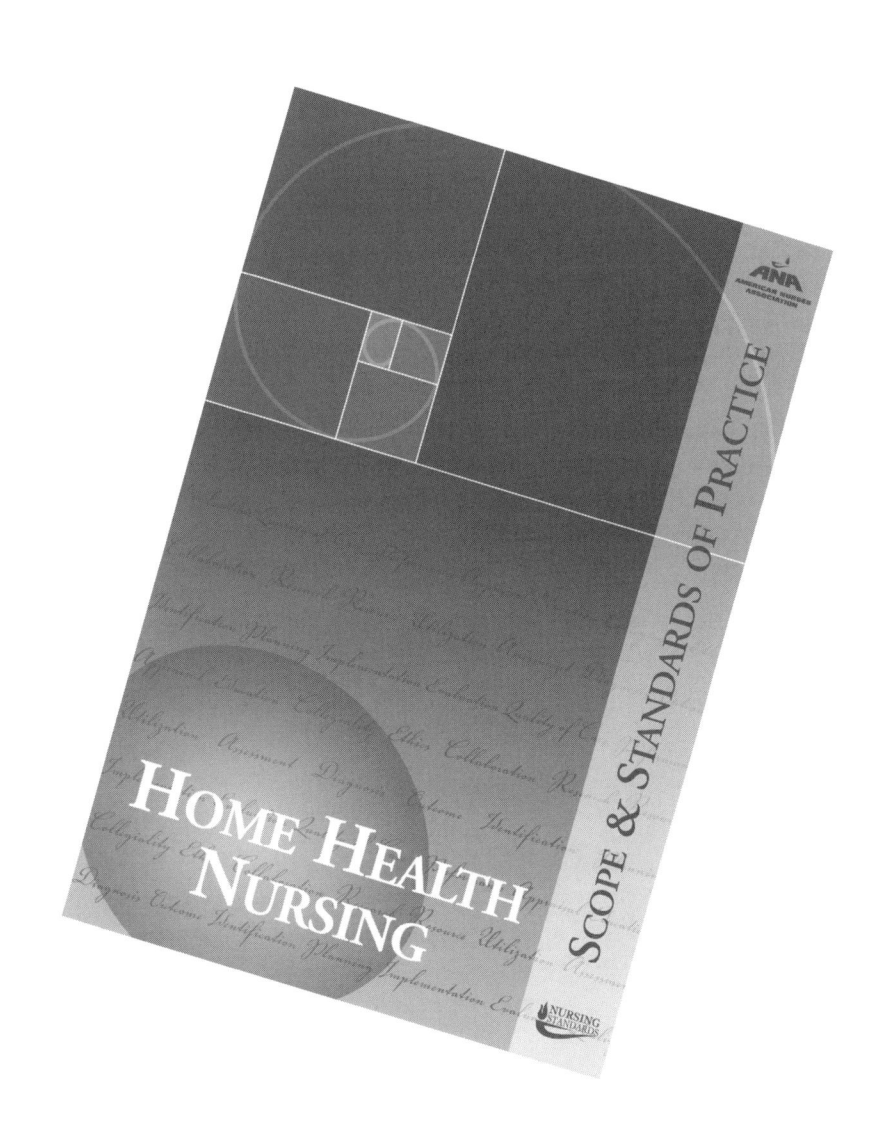

APPENDIX A. HOME HEALTH NURSING: SCOPE & STANDARDS OF PRACTICE (2007)

The content in this appendix is not current and is of historical significance only.

ACKNOWLEDGMENTS

The work group that created this 2007 revision of *Home Health Nursing: Scope and Standards of Practice* gratefully acknowledges the work of previous task forces in 1999, 1992, and 1986 to initiate the original documents on home health care.

Work Group Members (2007)

Marilyn D. Harris, MSN, RN, CNAA-BC, FAAN, Chair
Laura Beth Brown, MSN, C, RN
Joann K. Erb, PhD, RN
Soozi Flannigan, MSN, RN, APRN
Lisa A. Gorski, MS, APRN-BC, CRNI, FAAN
Carolyn J. Humphrey, MS, RN, FAAN
Patricia M. Hunt, MS, RN
Deana M. Kilmer, MBA, BS, RN
N. Jean Macdonald, MS, RN
Karen S. Martin, MSN, RN, FAAN
Paula Milone-Nuzzo, PhD, RN, FAAN, FHHC
Mary Narayan, MSN, APRN-BC, CTN
Mary St. Pierre, MSN, RN, MGA
Jeanie Stoker, MPA, RN-BC
Cynthia Struk, PhD, RN, PNP
Denise Swegles, BSN, RN, CHA

ANA Staff

Carol J. Bickford, PhD, RN-BC—Content editor
Patricia Rowell, PhD, APRN-BC—Content editor
Yvonne D. Humes, MSA—Project coordinator
Therese Myers, JD—Legal counsel

APPENDIX A. HOME HEALTH NURSING: SCOPE & STANDARDS OF PRACTICE (2007)

The content in this appendix is not current and is of historical significance only.

Contents

Acknowledgments	iii
Preface	vii
Home Health Nursing Scope of Practice	1
Evolution of Home Health Nursing	1
Definition of Home Health Nursing	2
Distinguishing Characteristics of Home Health Nursing	3
The Nursing Process in Home Health Nursing	4
Assessment	4
Diagnosis	5
Outcomes Identification	5
Planning	5
Implementation	6
Evaluation	7
Educational Preparation of Home Health Nurses	7
Home Health Nurse: Generalist	7
Home Health Nurse: Advanced Practice	9
Clinical Nurse Specialist	9
Nurse Practitioner	10
Roles of the Home Health Nurse	10
Care Manager and Coordinator of Care	11
Educator	12
Advocate	12
Administrator	14
Supervisor	14
Quality Improvement Expert	14
Trends, Issues, and Opportunities	15
Practice Issues	15
Clinical Concerns	15
Ethics	17
Legislation, Regulations, Legal Obligations, and Licensure	18
Legislation	18
Regulations	19
Legal Obligations and Licensure	19

APPENDIX A. HOME HEALTH NURSING: SCOPE & STANDARDS OF PRACTICE (2007)

The content in this appendix is not current and is of historical significance only.

The Nursing Shortage	20
Standardized Terminologies and Outcomes Management	20
Information Technology and Telehealth	22
Research	25
Summary	28
Standards of Home Health Nursing Practice	**29**
Standards of Practice	**29**
Standard 1. Assessment	29
Standard 2. Diagnosis	30
Standard 3. Outcomes Identification	31
Standard 4. Planning	33
Standard 5. Implementation	34
Standard 5a. Coordination of Care	35
Standard 5b. Health Teaching and Health Promotion	36
Standard 5c. Consultation	37
Standard 5d. Prescriptive Authority and Treatment	38
Standard 6. Evaluation	39
Standards of Professional Performance	**41**
Standard 7. Quality of Practice	41
Standard 8. Education	43
Standard 9. Professional Practice Evaluation	44
Standard 10. Collegiality	45
Standard 11. Collaboration	46
Standard 12. Ethics	47
Standard 13. Research	48
Standard 14. Resource Utilization	49
Standard 15. Leadership	50
Glossary	**53**
References	**57**
Bibliography	**63**
Appendix A. *Scope and Standards of Home Health Nursing Practice* **(1999)**	**65**
Index	**97**

APPENDIX A. HOME HEALTH NURSING: SCOPE & STANDARDS OF PRACTICE (2007)

The content in this appendix is not current and is of historical significance only.

PREFACE

Home Health Nursing: Scope and Standards of Practice describes the professional practice of all home health registered nurses. This scope statement and these updated standards of home health nursing practice are meant to guide, define, and direct home health professional nursing practice.

The American Nurses Association (ANA) has been active in the development of scope of practice and standards since the late 1960s. ANA published the first standards (*Standards of Nursing Practice*) for the nursing profession in 1973 (included in ANA, 2004). These standards were generic in nature and focused on the basic nursing process—a critical thinking model applicable to all registered nurses—composed of assessment, diagnosis, outcomes identification, planning, implementation, and evaluation (ANA, 2005, p.10; ANA, 2004, p. 3). Various revisions have ensued, the most recent being *Nursing: Scope and Standards of Practice (ANA, 2004)*, which is to be used in conjunction with *Nursing's Social Policy Statement, 2nd Edition* (ANA, 2003) and *Code of Ethics for Nurses with Interpretive Statements* (ANA, 2001). These three resources provide a complete and definitive description for better understanding of nursing practice and nursing's accountability to the public in the United States (ANA, 2004, p. *vi*).

Specialty nursing organizations have affirmed the 2004 ANA publication by using the template language of the standards when developing scope of practice statements and standards of practice for registered nurses in specialty practice. ANA published the first *Standards of Home Health Nursing Practice* in 1986; a revision followed in 1992. The 1999 revision, *Scope and Standards of Home Health Nursing Practice*, included a scope of practice statement to describe the specialty practice as well as its revised standards of practice. This latest revision (2007) includes a contemporary scope of practice statement and accompanying standards of practice to guide home health nursing practice today and in the future.

As part of its regular process of development, review, and maintenance of scope and standards of nursing practice, ANA convened a volunteer work group of home health nursing professionals in 2005 to review and revise the 1999 standards to best reflect contemporary home health nursing practice and provide a framework for future practice.

APPENDIX A. HOME HEALTH NURSING: SCOPE & STANDARDS OF PRACTICE (2007)

The content in this appendix is not current and is of historical significance only.

Registered nurses in different home health settings and in various roles responded to ANA's call for volunteers. They have worked on the document in small groups and through monthly conference calls since September 2005. The work group:

- assessed research reports, publications, and evidence-based practice;
- distributed and sought input on the updated draft scope and standards from nurses who attended the Home Healthcare Nurses Association (HHNA) meetings at the National Association for Home Care and Hospice (NAHC) annual meetings in October 2005 and 2006;
- shared information and requested input from nurses through a guest editorial in *Home Healthcare Nurse* (Harris, 2006);
- notified ANA's Constituent Member Associations (CMAs), specialty nursing organizations, home health organizations, and other stakeholders that input was requested on the document; and
- posted the draft document on ANA's Web site for public review and comment by interested nurses and others.

All public comments and suggestions were considered by the work group in preparing the final document. Reviews by the Committee on Nursing Practice Standards and Guidelines of the ANA Congress on Nursing Practice and Economics culminated in the final edits, acknowledgment of the scope of practice, approval of the standards of practice, and publication of this, the 2008 updated edition, *Home Health Nursing: Scope and Standards of Practice*.

The profession must incorporate the updated content on these pages into home health nursing practice across the country. The goal is to improve the health, well-being, and quality of life of all home healthcare patients and their families and other caregivers. This can best be accomplished through the significant and visible contributions of registered nurses using standards-based practice.

APPENDIX A. HOME HEALTH NURSING: SCOPE & STANDARDS OF PRACTICE (2007)

The content in this appendix is not current and is of historical significance only.

HOME HEALTH NURSING SCOPE OF PRACTICE

Evolution of Home Health Nursing

The specialty of home health nursing is rapidly growing and evolving because of demographic changes and technological advances. While community-based care has been provided for centuries, Florence Nightingale, William Rathbone, and their colleagues formalized the practice during the 1800s. The titles they selected—district nurses (home health) and health visitors (public health)—are still in use in the United Kingdom.

During the late nineteenth and early twentieth centuries, home health nursing services were organized in many cities and towns in the United States. Frequently, women from wealthy families provided the leadership and resources to establish nursing services. Although few of the women were nurses, they were genuinely concerned about local health and social issues.

Early nurse leaders, including Lillian Wald, Lavinia Dock, Margaret Sanger, and Mary Breckinridge, refined and publicized models of health promotion and disease prevention. In the late 1800s Visiting Nurse Associations (VNAs) and the nursing divisions of governmental health agencies, such as city and county health departments, provided the majority of services. Community health nurses, as generalists, gave nursing care to the sick as well as health promotion services to individuals, families, and communities. Public health principles and practice, and components of family and community care, were integrated into home-based nursing services.

Several key events drove the steady but slow growth of home care in the early 1900s. In 1909, the Metropolitan Life Insurance Company paid for nurses to care for their policyholders in the home. During World War II, as physicians made fewer home visits and focused instead on offices and hospitals, the home care movement grew, with nurses providing most of the health and illness care services in the home. In 1946, Montefiore Hospital in New York City developed a post-hospital acute care program and initiated convalescent home care.

In 1952, the American Nurses Association (ANA) and the National League for Nursing (NLN) became the primary national nursing organizations following the merger and restructuring of other organizations.

APPENDIX A. HOME HEALTH NURSING: SCOPE & STANDARDS OF PRACTICE (2007)

The content in this appendix is not current and is of historical significance only.

The NLN became the primary organization for the home health nursing specialty for the next 30 years.

The Medicare legislation of 1965, which included a home health benefit, increased the reach and visibility of home care and led to its significant growth. Because of the new reimbursement benefits, physicians and hospitals began to discharge patients earlier. New treatments and technology enabled more patients to be treated at home, resulting in increased referrals to existing agencies and the establishment of many new agencies, some affiliated with hospitals and some independent, commercial enterprises. Home health nursing practice emphasized acute care in the home, and some agencies began to offer services 24 hours a day, 7 days a week. In addition, the new legislation prompted organizational mergers, including the establishment of the Visiting Nurse Associations of America (VNAA) and the National Association for Home Care (NAHC) in 1982. These two organizations became the primary specialty organizations for home health nurses and continue to provide strong national leadership.

In the early 1980s diagnosis-related groups (DRGs) were phased in over a four-year period in hospitals nationwide. Implementation of the DRG system resulted in shorter hospital stays and increased use of home care services. Home health nurses were faced with providing highly complex clinical care to patients in their homes.

Responding to the expansion of nursing services provided in the home and the need to formalize this specialty practice, ANA published the first version of its practice standards, *Standards of Home Health Nursing Practice*, in 1986. Revised in 1992, this publication was followed by an expanded *Scope and Standards of Home Health Nursing Practice* in 1999.

At the beginning of the twenty-first century, home health nurses provide skilled care in the home that was not anticipated a few years ago. In addition, as a result of pandemic warnings and natural and man-made disasters, the home and community are increasing in importance as the recommended point of care delivery. In the future, home health nurses may be called upon to coordinate and deliver care unlike ever before.

Definition of Home Health Nursing

Home health nursing is the provision of nursing care to acutely ill, chronically ill, terminally ill, and well patients of all ages in

APPENDIX A. HOME HEALTH NURSING: SCOPE & STANDARDS OF PRACTICE (2007)

The content in this appendix is not current and is of historical significance only.

their residences. Home health nursing focuses on health promotion and care of the sick while integrating environmental, psychosocial, economic, cultural, and personal health factors affecting an individual's and family's health status (Humphrey & Milone-Nuzzo, 1996–1999, 2008).

Home health nursing is nursing practice applied to patients of all ages in the patients' residences, which may include private homes, assisted living, or personal care facilities. Although there are multiple ways to describe the recipient of home health care—patient, client, customer, and healthcare consumer—this document uses the term *patient*. Patients and their families and other caregivers are the focus of home health nursing practice. The goal of care is to maintain or improve the quality of life for patients and their families and other caregivers, or to support patients in their transition to end of life. This is accomplished through the initiation, coordination, management, and evaluation of resources needed to promote the patient's optimal level of well-being and function. Nursing activities necessary to achieve this goal may include preventive, maintenance, restorative, and rehabilitative interventions to manage existing health problems and prevent potential problems.

Although the term "home care" is used by many national associations and publications, the professional title of home health nurse is defined and recognized by the nursing profession, other healthcare professionals, and the public. The work group members involved in this scope and standards revision considered the terms "home care nurse" and "home health care nurse" and concluded that the title and tradition of *home health nurse* should be continued.

Distinguishing Characteristics of Home Health Nursing

Home health nursing is a specialized area of community health nursing practice which focuses on individuals in need of care in their homes, their families, and their caregivers. Home health nurses provide care to patients across the life span, from the pre-natal through the post-death periods. Home health nursing stresses the holistic management of personal health practices for the treatment of diseases or disability. Practice embraces primary, secondary, and tertiary prevention; assistance to families with coordination of community resources and health insurance benefits; and delivery of healthcare services in a patient's home, including non-conventional residences.

APPENDIX A. HOME HEALTH NURSING: SCOPE & STANDARDS OF PRACTICE (2007)

The content in this appendix is not current and is of historical significance only.

Home health reflects more than a change in location or acute care delivered in the home. Home health requires a change in the definition and structures of care to reflect a broad array of coordinated services, benefits, and caregivers available to patients experiencing complex problems. Home health nurses, who care for these patients, practice independently and require highly developed skills in assessment and care coordination. Although they practice in collaboration with other healthcare professionals, they most often are the only professionals in the home providing care to the patient. As such, they must be expert in assessment, clinical decision-making, and clinical practice. These skills form the foundation for planning, nursing care interventions, communication with other healthcare providers, and referral to other healthcare settings when appropriate.

Home health patients may require nursing care resources 24 hours a day, 7 days a week. The frequency and duration of these services is dependent upon the home care delivery model and holistic needs of the unit that is the patient and the family and other caregivers, ranging from intermittent visits to full-time extended daily care.

Home health nursing differs from other nursing specialties in the degree of responsibility nurses assume in managing the financial cost of care. Home health nurses work directly with public and private payers and with consumer-directed payment programs. Home health nurses must have advanced knowledge of reimbursement systems to help patients obtain the care they need while containing the cost of care.

The Nursing Process in Home Health Nursing

Home health nurses use the nursing process, the essential methodology by which patient goals are identified and achieved. The nursing process is comprised of assessment, diagnosis, outcomes identification, planning, implementation, and evaluation.

Assessment

Home health nurses assess the physical, psychosocial, and environmental factors that affect a patient's health to develop a comprehensive nursing care plan which will attain the patient's desired health outcomes in a culturally comfortable way. Physical assessment includes systems assessment, impact of the disease or condition on the patient, and monitoring of medications and therapies. Psychosocial assessment includes family, cultural, and spiritual assessments. Environmental assessment includes assessing the patient's safety, ability to meet daily needs, and ability to participate in meaningful activities in the home. In the home setting, understanding the influences of family dynamics and the home environment on the physical and emotional state of the patient is essential for effective care management.

Diagnosis

Home health nurses derive their diagnoses from the assessment data. Diagnoses can be focused on the physical, psychosocial, cultural, spiritual, environmental, economic, and interpersonal aspects of care. Home health nurses, in collaboration with the patient, the family, and other caregivers, identify actual nursing problems as well as situations that might become problems if unattended. Diagnoses may be specific to nursing practice or may require the home health nurse to serve as a care manager with other members of the interdisciplinary care team.

Outcomes Identification

The home health nurse works with the patient, the family, and other caregivers to identify attainable and measurable goals for the patient based on the patient's medical and nursing diagnoses. These goals are the patient outcomes expected as a result of the care the home health nurse and the interdisciplinary team provide. Optimal health and well-being, effective self-management of health problems, or a peaceful death are examples of expected outcomes.

Planning

Home health nurses plan care in collaboration with the patient, family and other caregivers, and other healthcare providers, to develop interventions that are incorporated in the patient's care plan. When the patient receives services from multiple practitioners, including non-professionals, home health nurses often assume the role of care manager and coordinate all the involved disciplines, including the patient's primary care provider and other caregivers, to optimize patient outcomes.

The home health nurse provides clinical supervision to Licensed Practical/Vocational Nurses (LPN/LVN) and home health aides in accordance with the Medicare Conditions of Participation (COPs) and state practice standards. According to a 2002 study (Stoker, 2003), all 50 states allow LPN/LVNs to provide home care under the direct and indirect supervision of an RN. As a home health nurse, the RN must be aware of the responsibility in the supervision and delegation processes as defined by the profession, state practice acts, accrediting bodies, and agency policy.

Implementation

Home health nurses provide skilled nursing interventions to patients and their families and caregivers, including teaching, counseling, care management, resource coordination, and evaluative data collection. In collaboration with the patient, the family, and other caregivers, home health nurses determine the most appropriate nursing care strategies to meet identified patient outcomes, which often include complementary and cultural therapies.

Patient and family and other caregiver teaching is integral to the role of home health nurses. Teaching supports the achievement of patient outcomes and the movement of the patient and the family toward independence. As expert patient educators, home health nurses use a variety of media and strategies to develop and reinforce enhanced self-care skills. Home health nurses share knowledge of community health resources with the patient, the family, and other caregivers. Through this information exchange and advocacy, home health nurses encourage patients, families, and other caregivers to plan for and seek additional services as their needs dictate.

One of the primary responsibilities of home health nurses is patient advocacy. This is incorporated in all phases of the nursing process, not just during implementation of the plan of care and associated therapies. Patient advocacy includes assisting patients in navigating the healthcare delivery system, supporting them in making healthcare decisions, and helping them access community resources to support independence. Informing, supporting, and affirming that the decision-making of patients, their families, and other caregivers are important adjuncts to achieving patient care objectives and patient goals.

The home health nurse will also assess the implementation of the care plan and care provided by the LPN/LVN and home health aide. While the LPN/LVN and home health aide may be team members in the home health setting, the RN must provide ongoing assessment and supervision as required by the law to help ensure positive outcomes.

APPENDIX A. HOME HEALTH NURSING: SCOPE & STANDARDS OF PRACTICE (2007)

The content in this appendix is not current and is of historical significance only.

Home health nursing is provided in the context of a highly differentiated and complex healthcare delivery system and requires special time management and organizational skills. To help patients achieve desired health outcomes, home health nurses need specific knowledge about the dynamic financial and regulatory aspects of care that are unique to this practice.

Evaluation

The evaluation of patient outcomes provides critical data to determine the effectiveness of nursing care. Home health nurses must critically evaluate their practice through quality improvement activities, critical incident reviews, and participation in research.

Educational Preparation of Home Health Nurses

Home health nursing, because of its level of independence in practice, requires a high degree of knowledge and expertise. Although baccalaureate nurses are better prepared to meet the demands of home health nursing practice, nurses with associate degrees or diplomas can enter home health nursing as members of the nursing team. All nurses who enter home health nursing are expected to grow in their ability to assume home health nursing's roles and demands through the support of their colleagues, structured preceptor programs, clinical experiences, and lifelong learning through academic and continuing education. At this time certification as a home health nurse is not available. However, home health nurses can affirm their knowledge and skills through other applicable nursing certification in such areas as pediatrics, critical care, hospice and palliative care, and gerontological nursing.

Home Health Nurse: Generalist

Home health nurses provide all aspects of nursing care in accord with *Nursing: Scope and Standards of Practice* (ANA, 2004), as well as the more detailed home health nursing standards. Competent home health nursing practice requires flexibility, creativity, and innovative approaches to situations and problems in the context of individual and environmental differences and widely varying resource availability.

APPENDIX A. HOME HEALTH NURSING: SCOPE & STANDARDS OF PRACTICE (2007)

The content in this appendix is not current and is of historical significance only.

Effective home health nursing practice includes identification of and attention to environmental, economic, familial, and cultural differences. In addition, a basic understanding of psychosocial and safety issues affecting patients, their families, and other caregivers is critical for the effective delivery of home health nursing. Because patients residing in their homes may receive healthcare services from an array of providers, home health nurses must assume the role of care manager and coordinator.

Therefore, the preferred minimum qualifications for a registered nurse practicing in the home health setting are:

- A baccalaureate degree in nursing.
- Ability to incorporate communication and motivation skills and principles in the home health setting.
- Ability to apply critical thinking to physical, psychosocial, environmental, cultural, family, and safety issues.
- Ability to utilize clinical decision-making in applying the nursing process to patients in their places of residence.
- Ability to practice as an effective member of an interdisciplinary team.
- Competency in applying care management skills.

Home health nursing is an autonomous practice requiring knowledge and skills often not attained in basic nursing educational programs or other practice settings. Therefore, all registered nurses (RN) must be initially assessed for their ability to apply the nursing process to the home health setting, including consideration of prior home care and general nursing practice experience and educational preparation.

The necessary knowledge base and skills for home health nursing can be developed through formal orientation programs, structured preceptor programs, and guided clinical experience based on the specific learning needs of the nurse. Each home health nurse must build and maintain the professional knowledge, skills, and abilities that support evidence-based practice and clinical decision-making that empowers the patient to attain self-management and achieve the best outcomes possible. The employing agency also has an obligation to establish an environment conducive to such professional development.

APPENDIX A. HOME HEALTH NURSING: SCOPE & STANDARDS OF PRACTICE (2007)

The content in this appendix is not current and is of historical significance only.

Home Health Nurse: Advanced Practice

Advanced practice registered nurses (APRN) working in home health settings possess advanced specialized clinical knowledge and skills to provide health care to patients, families, and groups in their places of residence. The Clinical Nurse Specialist (CNS) and Nurse Practitioner (NP) are the advanced practice RNs who most frequently practice in home health.

The increasingly older and chronically ill home health patient population requires a high level of clinical expertise as treatment and medication regimens have grown in complexity. These patient characteristics, combined with the pressure to improve clinical outcomes, require more advanced practice nurses in home health.

Advanced practice registered nurses hold a master's or doctoral degree in nursing. They build on the practice of registered nurses by demonstrating a greater depth and breadth of knowledge, a greater synthesis of data, increased complexity of skills and interventions, and significant role autonomy (ANA, 2004, p.14). The APRN in home health settings evaluates and implements evidence-based practice to improve care for patients and families, develops specialized programs that promote improvement in clinical outcomes, collaborates with community resources, and may participate in research pertaining to home health nursing practice and home health services.

APRNs may prescribe pharmacologic and non-pharmacologic treatments in the direct management of acute and chronic illness and disease in compliance with federal and state regulations in the home health setting. APRNs are specially suited to the development and management of outcomes-based research in the area of home care. The APRN may also assume the role of nurse educator and mentor undergraduate nursing students and graduate level practitioners in home health practice.

Clinical Nurse Specialist

The CNS is an expert in evidence-based nursing practice, treating and managing the health concerns of patients, families, and populations. CNS practice is targeted toward achieving quality, cost-effective outcomes in accordance with three spheres of influence (NACNS, 2004):

- *Patient care* – Comprehensive assessment, expert care and care planning, care management for home health patients, families, and groups with specific or complex needs, and application of evidence-based clinical interventions for patient populations with similar needs or disease states.
- *Nurses and nursing practice* – Meeting the educational needs of nurses through formal and informal methods, promoting evidence-based practice to achieve clinical outcomes, acting as a consultant to staff and administration in the area of improving clinical outcomes.
- *Organization or system* – Initiating change and continuous improvement to benefit the system, developing and implementing evidence-based, best practice models, development of programs for groups of patients that enhance patient outcomes.

Nurse Practitioner

Nurse practitioners (NPs) perform comprehensive assessments, diagnose and treat actual and potential health problems, manage acute and chronic illness, and promote health and the prevention of illness and injury. They diagnose, develop differential diagnoses, and conduct, supervise, and interpret diagnostic and laboratory tests. NPs oversee, manage care, and direct the delivery of clinical services within an integrated system of health care using the transitional and palliative care approaches, thus allowing for continuity of care to and from all settings (home, institution, and community). NPs practice autonomously and in collaboration with other healthcare professionals to treat and manage patients' health problems, and serve as researchers, consultants, and patient advocates for individuals, families, groups, and communities. NPs expand access to services and improve quality of care for patients with advanced chronic illness while improving cost effectiveness.

Roles of the Home Health Nurse

The home health nursing roles detailed below cover: care management and coordination of care, education, advocacy, administration, supervision, and quality improvement.

APPENDIX A. HOME HEALTH NURSING: SCOPE & STANDARDS OF PRACTICE (2007)

The content in this appendix is not current and is of historical significance only.

Care Manager and Coordinator of Care

This role involves not only the delivery of direct care to the patient but also coordination of care provided by other disciplines. When a patient is admitted to service, the nurse care manager uses the nursing process to assess the patient's unique situation, and develops a Plan of Care (POC) in consultation with the patient and the physician. The home health nurse implements the POC to help the patient reach maximal potential and evaluates the outcomes. Specific activities in this process include:

- Performs a comprehensive holistic assessment using the patient, family and other caregivers, and other pertinent sources of information about the patient.

- Designs the POC considering the patient's unique strengths and limitations, and the impact of cultural and religious beliefs on the patient's cognitive, physical, and emotional condition.

- Prioritizes care based on mutual goal setting and outcome identification by the patient and the nurse.

- Provides accurate documentation to support initiation and continuation of skilled services.

- Provides direct care to patients including ongoing assessment of condition, education of the patient and the family, evaluation of effectiveness of care, and revision of POC to achieve the patient's optimal health potential.

- Delegates care to nurses, nursing students, licensed practical nurses (LPNs), and home health aides (HHAs) utilizing the principles of delegation. Provides ongoing instruction and supervision.

- Determines the appropriate utilization of services, acknowledging financial parameters, while developing and implementing a POC that promotes optimal patient outcomes.

- Evaluates the effectiveness of care and the progress of the patient toward goals and revises the plan as needed to help the patient achieve maximal potential and positive outcomes, which may include dying with dignity.

- Collaborates with the interdisciplinary team and maintains communication related to the patient's response to the POC.

- Collaborates with the healthcare providers by communicating changes in condition and progress toward goal attainment.

Educator

Home health nurses educate patients, families and other caregivers, and the community. A major responsibility of home health nurses is to provide instruction to patients, families, and other caregivers on acute and chronic disease processes, and to help patients develop other self-management skills and abilities. In this role, nurses provide information, demonstrate techniques, and evaluate performance of procedures by patients, families, and other caregivers. Nurses must be able to identify barriers to learning, provide instructions using a variety of methods, and incorporate health beliefs and cultural and religious practices into the process of patient education. The home health nurse also:

- Educates patients, families, and other caregivers on healthy lifestyle, health promotion, and disease prevention.
- Provides information and education concerning reimbursement for home care services.

Nurses may also conduct community education programs and provide information about available home health services and reimbursement for care. Home health nurses educate physicians and other health professionals about opportunities to work collaboratively in the home setting. The goals for collaboration include helping the patient achieve optimal function, maintain independence, and in some cases helping terminally ill patients remain at home.

Advocate

The home health nurse is often the health professional who interacts most with patients, their families, and other caregivers. As a result of this interaction, nurses frequently become aware of problems or circumstances that interfere with a patient's recovery, safety, or well-being. Home health nurses treat the individual in a holistic manner and recognize when additional clarification or support is needed or additional resources are required. Nurses may also identify factors that interfere with a patient's recovery, safety, or adherence to the treatment plan. As advocates, home health nurses serve as a liaison between the patient, the family (as providers of care), healthcare provider, and the healthcare system; provide information to assist in informed decision-making; and support decisions that a patient makes. The home health nurse also:

- Identifies and coordinates community resources to assist patients in achieving maximum health potential.
- Empowers patients and families in their interactions with the healthcare system by providing information and support.
- Provides information about care options, reimbursement, and community resources.
- Implements programs, such as medication reconciliation and fall prevention, to maximize patient safety.
- Refers the patient to community services and resources to ensure continuity of care after discharge from home care.
- Promotes continuity of care through collaboration within the agency and with other healthcare providers.

The home health nurse is also accountable for advocacy for both professional development and the professional practice of home health nursing. The responsibilities include ongoing education, mentoring, contributing to the ongoing development of the practice through active participation in professional membership, promoting the image of professional home health nursing, and actively participating in legislation and research that affect home health nursing. Other professional advocacy responsibilities include:

- Acting as a role model for professional nursing and as a proactive nursing advocate.
- Supporting and encouraging others to study and practice nursing.
- Sharing knowledge and experience with colleagues within and outside of home health.
- Serving as a leader in health promotion and patient care by advancing one's own knowledge base.
- Incorporating concepts of evidence-based practice in planning nursing interventions.
- Fostering cohesive relationships and collaborating with all members of the nursing profession.

- Maintaining membership and active involvement in professional organizations to remain current in health policy that impacts practice.
- Participating in formal quality assessment and improvement activities.

Administrator

The home health administrator is responsible for maintaining quality care in a dynamic environment in which reimbursement requirements, accreditation standards, and healthcare systems change frequently. The administrator provides leadership to meet these challenges and ensure availability of competent, qualified staff. The administrator must be knowledgeable about computerization, financial issues, documentation, and new opportunities while maintaining organizational and patient care standards. As the conscience of the organization, the administrator concentrates on the mission of the organization and its first priority, namely the patient and the patient's needs. The administrator also serves as a liaison between staff and outside agencies, including national and legal entities. The administrator speaks for home health staff and patients and brings attention to problems and limitations of the present system.

Supervisor

The home health supervisor, or clinical manager, is responsible for the coordination and evaluation of patient care activities. The supervisor facilitates the professional development of home health nurses by providing education and support in clinical decision-making, disease management, and compliance with regulations related to home health services. The supervisor supports achievement of the organization's mission and goals by ensuring the availability of a competent nursing staff.

Quality Improvement Expert

The nurse leader who is responsible for quality improvement promotes excellence in clinical practice in the organization. This includes the collection and analysis of quantitative and qualitative data to evaluate patients' responses to care. The nurse evaluates the organization's processes and structure to ensure quality care and incorporates scientific evidence into policies, procedures, and practices. The nurse also provides education and support and may mentor new staff or supervisors. This role includes translating and disseminating quality data to appropriate stakeholders.

Trends, Issues, and Opportunities

Home health nurses, their organizations, and the healthcare industry face exciting, although sobering, trends, issues, and opportunities. Woven throughout this section are comments about the need for home health nurses and their organizations to:

- Acknowledge the development of health consumerism and increased partnerships with individuals, families, and communities.
- Recognize changing demographics related to aging, chronic illness, and cultural diversity.
- Collaborate with other healthcare professionals and providers.
- Become active change agents rather than reactive participants.
- Note the dramatic impacts of globalization.
- Prepare for the future.

Trends, issues, and opportunities influence the role of today's home health nurse and are likely to do so even more during the next 10 to 20 years.

Practice Issues

Clinical Concerns

Medicare remains the largest single payer of home care: 69% of home care patients are over 65 years old (NAHC, 2004). Chronic illnesses are increasingly common among older adults and account for the majority of home health diagnoses. Chronic illnesses are also costly, accounting for more than 70% of the cost of health care in the United States each year (CDC, 2004). Chronically ill patients frequently require multiple medications, ongoing treatment, and monitoring. The impact on quality of life and functional ability is significant. Many patients with chronic illnesses that require lifestyle modification as part of their care plan do not adhere to such recommendations to manage their illnesses. With an increasing emphasis on healthcare outcomes, home health nurses are challenged to work more effectively with the chronically ill.

The World Health Organization (2003) emphasizes that working with patients to improve adherence to treatment and medication protocols is of critical importance to patient safety, overall health, and reducing the cost of health care. Home health nurses must rise to the challenge of identifying barriers to adherence and helping patients self-manage their illnesses. Home health nurses must work collaboratively with patients and families to set realistic healthcare goals, adopt problem-solving skills, manage symptoms, and reduce the risk for disease exacerbation.

Home health clinical practice continues to include care of acutely ill patients, allowing for early discharge of hospitalized patients to receive more complex treatments such as advanced wound care treatments and infusion therapies at home. With improved drug therapies and home monitoring capabilities, some patients with diagnoses such as infections and deep vein thrombosis can be treated at home without hospitalization. When managing acute conditions in the home setting, the safety of the home environment is essential in relation to both the types of treatments provided and the presence of caregiver support.

While home health nurses must function as generalists caring for a wide variety of patients and conditions, increasingly there will be an emphasis on specialty areas of expertise. For example, there is growing interest in providing palliative care and behavioral health programs in the home health environment. Home health programs for prevalent diagnoses such as heart failure or diabetes, promotion of specialized home health nursing skills, and use of advanced practice nurses are increasingly cited as effective home health strategies associated with improved clinical outcomes.

For home health nurses, one goal has always been to help patients remain healthy and avoid acute care hospitalization. This outcome has become a focus of national concern as hospitalization contributes to the ever increasing risk and cost of health care. In a recent study, a number of strategies were identified as important to reducing hospitalization among home health patients including clinical strategies of preventing falls, medication management, case management, patient and caregiver education, and disease management programs (NAHC, 2006).

APPENDIX A. HOME HEALTH NURSING: SCOPE & STANDARDS OF PRACTICE (2007)

The content in this appendix is not current and is of historical significance only.

Home health agencies are responding to an environment of consumerism by better defining their services and developing new services to meet the needs of the community and healthcare payers. This consumer focus helps ensure that home health services promote wellness, especially among high-risk patients living in the community. Examples include fall prevention, medication safety, pain management, education related to infection prevention, and immunization programs.

The ability to measure and compare outcomes using Outcome Assessment and Information Set (OASIS) data has had a major impact on home health nursing. As home health evolves into a pay-for-performance model of reimbursement, home health nurses will become better educated about and accountable to achieving positive patient outcomes. Home health nurses must use effective strategies to provide home health care with attention to age and developmental stages, cultural issues, and evidence-based practices.

The steep increase in the older adult population, the rising prevalence of chronic illnesses, and the challenges of cultural diversity will significantly affect home health practice in the future. Home health services will become an even more critical element of the healthcare system by controlling the overall cost of healthcare, keeping patients out of expensive acute care hospitals, and reducing the need for patients to reside in long-term care facilities.

Ethics

In the general world of health care, the patient is the "outsider" and is expected to behave according to the "rules" of the hospital, outpatient setting, or physician office. Home health care is unique because the home health nurse is the "outsider" with the patient, family, and other caregivers "allowing" the nurse to provide care in their home. Home health nurses provide care in settings ranging from the most luxurious mansions to tents under a bridge. They recognize that patients' homes are their "castles" and the optimal places to educate and promote health.

Home health nurses may face numerous ethical issues during the course of care. The patient's privacy may be compromised as family members and caregivers are taught to provide care. Patients or family members or caregivers may fail to comply with healthcare recommendations such as treatments or medications. Care provided by family members or caregivers may be poor, even neglectful or abusive. Patients may choose to follow medical, nutritional, pharmacological, and other courses that are not within the plan of care or optimal to their health. Patients may require services beyond what the home health agency is able to provide or beyond what the insurance or other payer will cover. Physicians may order treatments that conflict with best practice. Challenges arise when home health nurses must balance patient needs with personal safety, such as animals or illegal activities in the home.

Home health nurses must explore their own personal values in relation to the rules and regulations that influence practice. *Code of Ethics for Nurses with Interpretive Statements* (ANA, 2001) provides guidance. The home health nurse acts as a patient advocate and maintains confidentiality, safety, security, dignity, and respect for both the patient and the family. Home health agencies must provide guidelines and resources for ethical issues that arise. Increasingly, home health agencies utilize interdisciplinary ethics committees to explore ethical issues and formulate plans to resolve such issues.

Legislation, Regulations, Legal Obligations, and Licensure

"Government's influence on professional practice, quality health care, and agency administration increases with each passing year. Federal, state, and local laws and regulations impact the day-to-day operations." (Mebus & Piskor, 2005, p. 675). It is important for home health nurses to understand how they can influence the legislative and regulatory processes, identify resources, and take action when necessary. Furthermore, they must be knowledgeable about and comply with existing statutes and regulations. Information about legislation, regulations, and legal matters is available from government agencies, such as the Centers for Medicare and Medicaid Services and state and local health departments, in government publications like the *Federal Register*, and through employers and professional and trade associations.

Legislation

Home health nurses have a responsibility to be aware of and seek to influence federal, state, and local legislation that affects the nursing profession. In addition, home health nurses should actively work to influence legislation that affects the delivery of healthcare services in the

APPENDIX A. HOME HEALTH NURSING: SCOPE & STANDARDS OF PRACTICE (2007)

The content in this appendix is not current and is of historical significance only.

home. These goals can be accomplished by monitoring professional and trade associations for information about congressional activities and state and local legislative initiatives, and by taking action to influence legislation through advocacy. Formal organizations, such as professional and trade associations, provide a variety of venues for legislative action.

Regulations

Home health nurses must be knowledgeable of federal, state, and local regulations that govern their practice, including nurse licensure requirements. In addition, they should be knowledgeable of and adhere to federal, state, and local quality, payment, and general health and hygiene regulations, and safe work practices. Ideally, home health nurses should participate in the regulatory process by taking an active role in such activities as government technical expert panels and submission of formal comments on proposed regulations.

Legal Obligations and Licensure

Legal obligations of home health nurses include compliance with existing statutes and regulations and avoidance of negligence and breach of contract. Legal requirements protect the rights of individuals, ensure fair business practices, impose a legal duty of care, and control fraudulent and abusive practices. The first step in meeting legal obligations is to have an adequate knowledge base. Therefore, home health nurses must first be familiar with federal, state, and local laws.

Home health nurses must adhere to individual professional licensure rules and organizational policies and procedures, which serve as the basis for standards for quantity and quality of care, breach of contract, and patient abandonment. They must know the content of the nurse practice acts for their work settings and understand the implications of the mutual recognition model of nurse licensure if it is applicable. Other patient-centered legal requirements that home health nurses must adhere to include federal, state, and local requirements for privacy and security of health information, civil rights, and the protection of individuals against abuse, neglect, and exploitation. In addition, home health nurses must comply with both state and federal false claims, anti-kickback, and physician self-referral laws and support their employers' compliance efforts. Failure to adhere to legal requirements can result in a wide range of penalties, ranging from disciplinary action against a nursing license and financial liability to criminal charges and exclusion from government programs.

The Nursing Shortage

In 2002 the Joint Commission (formerly the Joint Commission on Accreditation of Healthcare Organizations) reported over 126,000 nursing openings; some home health agencies were being forced to refuse new patients because of a shortfall in home health nurses (Huston, 2006). The gap between the demand for nurses and the supply will continue to grow exponentially. In fact, registered nurses are projected to compose the second largest number of new jobs among all occupations. Home healthcare employment is expected to increase rapidly because of the growing number of older persons with functional disabilities, consumer preference for care in the home, and technological advances that make it possible to bring increasingly complex treatments into the home. (U.S. Department of Labor and Statistics, 2006).

A recent study (Flynn, 2005) examined the factors that attract nurses to and that dissatify them in home health care. The factors that attract included practice flexibility, independence, and more time for direct patient contact that enabled the nurse to teach patients and families (Flynn, 2005). Paperwork and excessive documentation caused the most dissatisfaction; other common issues included overtime work, low salaries, weather, and wear and tear on the car. The increasing cost of transportation affects the entire country and is likely to further impede home health nursing recruitment and retention. Home health administrators are challenged to examine workplace issues such as personal safety and environment, and work with staff to make improvements needed to create attractive employment settings.

Standardized Terminologies and Outcomes Management

Standardized terminologies and outcomes management are mentioned regularly by the public media and payers and are included in most health-related publications and national and international conferences. These factors have an increasingly visible impact on practice, documentation, information management, and reimbursement of home health nurses, their agencies, and the healthcare industry. What works best?

APPENDIX A. HOME HEALTH NURSING: SCOPE & STANDARDS OF PRACTICE (2007)

The content in this appendix is not current and is of historical significance only.

Have patients improved? By how much? From what perspective? How much will it cost? According to Lang, "If we cannot name it, we cannot control it, finance it, teach it, research it, or put it into public policy" (Clark & Lang, 1992).

These questions and the attempts to provide answers are not new. In 1893, physician Jacques Bertillon led an international effort to create a system for statistically classifying the causes of death and disease. Adopted worldwide within a decade, this system led directly to the International Classification of Diseases (ICD) and a series of reference works still in use. The current tenth revision (ICD-10) is used by all member states of the World Health Organization (WHO, 2007). Florence Nightingale was the first nurse to consistently use the scientific method and to transform data into information. In the 1850s she gathered systematic data, transformed a hospital into an efficient institution within 2 months, documented evidence graphically, and publicized her results widely.

During the 1950s and 1960s, nursing leaders in the United States began to conduct evaluation research, explore the relationship of services to client outcomes, and focus on problems that arise with clients out of nursing diagnosis. Simultaneously, physicians advanced systems for nomenclature and classification, including the initial version of Systematized Nomenclature of Medicine (SNOMED). The First National Conference on Classification of Nursing Diagnoses was held in 1973, the same time that the Visiting Nurse Association of Omaha (Nebraska) began to standardize terms for client problems.

In 1989 ANA anticipated outcome management and electronic health record developments that would require standardized terminologies and databases and formed a committee to address these trends. In 1992, the committee recognized four interface terminologies that met selection criteria: NANDA (North American Nursing Diagnosis Association), Omaha System, Home Health Care Classification (HHCC), and Nursing Interventions Classification (NIC). Development and refinement have continued within nursing and other healthcare professions. A total of twelve terminologies and data element sets are currently recognized (ANA, 2006). The additional eight are: International Classification of Nursing Practice (ICNP); Nursing Outcomes Classification (NOC); Perioperative Nursing Data Set; Nursing Minimum Data Set; Nursing Management Minimum Data Set; ABC Codes; Logical Observation Identifiers, Names, and Codes (LOINC®); and SNOMED CT®. Many vendors are adding these terminologies to their software; some are evident to clinician users and others are not visible, such as reference terminologies.

Beginning in 1999, Medicare-certified home health agencies were required to use the Outcome and Assessment Information Set (OASIS), a nationwide attempt to quantify and track patient outcomes of care. Clinicians typically complete this assessment tool of more than 80 items for new patients admitted to home health services. Children and pregnant women are excluded. OASIS data must also be submitted at designated interim periods and at discharge from the home health agency.

Home health agencies participate in outcome-based quality improvement and related quality improvement and benchmarking activities. The Centers for Medicare and Medicaid Services (Centers) publish aggregate clinical data. The Centers indicate they will initiate a new program, "Pay for Performance," that will offer financial incentives for exceeding certain outcome levels and financial penalties for underachievement. Regardless of what the Centers introduces, third-party payers, accreditation and certification groups, private foundations, international governments, and consumers are applying increased pressure on healthcare providers to focus on standardization and outcomes management. Comparison of home health patients, nurses and their professional colleagues, and agencies is the present and the future.

Information Technology and Telehealth

Historically, home health nurses, their clinician colleagues, and their agencies have been innovators and early adopters of communication devices and technology (Rogers, 1995). Clinicians now consider cellular phones a necessity for organizing their schedules, contacting referral sources, and reporting visit findings. Nurses, their agencies, and their patients are now embracing computers, the Internet, and telehealth.

Few home health nurses used telehealth or personal computers in the 1990s because few vendors offered products designed for clinical use. The Internet was launched in 1992. Since 2000, personal, home health agency, and patient use of automation, the Internet, and telehealth have exploded nationally and globally. Many patients and their families use the Internet to become well informed about diagnoses, medications,

APPENDIX A. HOME HEALTH NURSING: SCOPE & STANDARDS OF PRACTICE (2007)

The content in this appendix is not current and is of historical significance only.

and treatment. Changes in Medicare regulations and reimbursement have encouraged agencies to invest in hardware and software. Increasingly, home health clinicians complete most of their documentation online for patients' electronic health records.

Many home health agencies have robust clinical, financial, scheduling, and statistical management information systems that are more user-friendly and integrated than their local hospitals' (Martin, 2005). An increasing number of home health agencies use telehealth. Huston (2006) states that as many as 45% of all home health episodes of care may be suitable for telehealth intervention. To understand the application of telehealth to home health nursing, it is important to define it. In its 2001 Report to Congress, the Department of Health and Human Services (2002) defined telehealth as the "use of telecommunication and information technologies to provide healthcare services at a distance to include diagnosis, treatment, public health, consumer health information, and health professions education." A more recent expanded definition (Brantley, Laney-Cummings, & Spivack, 2004) includes the integration of various applications such as clinical health delivery, management of healthcare information, education, and administrative services within a common infrastructure.

Telehealth within the framework of home health nursing can be broadly defined as the delivery of patient care services using technology to eliminate distance, time, or resource barriers in an effort to improve patient health outcomes. Technology applications include but are not limited to the following:

- Telemonitors with peripheral biometric attachments for remotely monitoring biophysical parameters such as weight or more complex measurement such as oxygen saturation or glucose levels.

- Phone technology with two-way connectivity which allows for monitoring of patient activity or response to disease management parameters such as pain, activity level, symptom exacerbation, diet, or behavioral cues. This information may be correlated with biophysical parameters.

- In-home message devices with disease management education, advice, and medication or treatment reminders with compliance monitoring features that may be remotely transmitted via phone or Internet technology or evaluated at nursing visits.

- Video cameras for monitoring all aspects of care delivery particularly focusing on wound management, home care aide supervision, or other aspects of clinical care usually necessitating direct observation.

- Personal computers with Internet connectivity for supervised communication, medical record access, or patient education.

- Video conferencing that allows nurses, physicians, and other healthcare providers to communicate about patient-specific care or to learn new disease management interventions.

Information technology and telehealth can lead to more effective and efficient communication that, in turn, can lead to enhanced quality of care, improved patient and clinician safety, and increased productivity. However, information technology and telehealth cannot replace the necessity or value of direct care. New technology does introduce tension in the workplace and may be threatening because it often represents a significant change, and requires education, financial resources, and new styles of operation (Bowles & Baugh, 2007).

The changes in information technology are dramatic and rapid at all levels in this country and globally. The changes will increasingly influence the practice of home health nurses. The federal government has established the Office of the National Coordinator for Health Information Technology (http://www.hhs.gov/healthit), whose agenda proposes that all documentation be converted to electronic systems in the near future. In addition to providers' electronic health records (EHR; see below), individuals could have microchips to store their own personal health data. Personal EHRs may become the norm rather than the exception in the near future.

The *electronic health record* is the longitudinal collection of a patient's personal and medical information stored in a computer-readable format. While it has been reported that less than 10% of hospitals in the United States have implemented their technology to include the EHR, home health agencies appear to be utilizing and embracing it. Since 2000, 63% of home health agencies have implemented some type of point-of-care technology (Utterback & Waldo, 2005) that includes various software, hardware, and EHR processes.

SNOMED CT®, LOINC®, and HL7 have been selected as the national standards for providers to link and exchange clinical data. While the governments of the United States and the United Kingdom initially agreed to mandate SNOMED CT, numerous other countries are joining the initiative. Individuals, groups, and countries with the most economic resources are not alone in the use of the Internet and information technology to obtain and communicate health-related information; it is ubiquitous. The regional health information organization (RHIO) effort is intended to encourage collaboration throughout the United States. Vendors are developing and producing smaller and faster digital and multifunctional devices. Web access is expected to replace current technology, and Web-based education is ubiquitous. Today's home health nurses will soon need to use new devices and methods that have not yet been invented. Home health nurses who anticipate and embrace technological developments have evidenced many positive outcomes for their patients.

Research

Diverse research that is pertinent to home health nursing practice includes single studies, studies conducted by members of other disciplines or interdisciplinary teams involving home health nurses, and programs of research. Schumacher and Marren (2004) note the increasing diversity, sophistication, and number of studies published in their extensive literature review. They group their review into five broad areas: nursing classification studies, critical transitions in the illness trajectory, family education and support, specific conditions prevalent in home care, and population diversity. Research priorities identified by Madigan and Vanderboom (2005) include outcomes, health policy, the use of advanced practice nurses, and models of care and best practice.

In general, the number of home health nurse researchers and the extent of funded home health studies are limited, especially in comparison to acute and long-term care research. However, the Centers for Medicare and Medicaid Services (CMS) has identified the reduction of the hospitalization rate of home health patients as a national priority. This emphasis has stimulated research on patient risk factors related to home care and interventions and strategies to reduce risk. A study of home health agencies with the lowest hospitalization rates was recently completed (NAHC, 2006). Fifteen agency strategies were identified as instrumental in preventing hospitalizations; these strategies included assessing and reducing the risks for falls, increasing home visit frequency at the start of care, and giving attention to organizational culture.

The content in this appendix is not current and is of historical significance only.

Evidence-based practice and evidence-based guidelines are important to home health nurses. Clinical practice guidelines developed by the University of Iowa School of Nursing (e.g., gerontological interventions) and the American Heart Association/American College of Cardiology (e.g., guidelines for heart failure management) are examples of such efforts. While the number of studies specific to home health and capable of serving as a foundation for evidence-based practice is still small, increasing interest will encourage expansion of the research base, increased opportunities for home health nurse researchers, more interdisciplinary collaboration, improved funding, and better client outcomes.

Programs of clinical and administrative research offer the greatest opportunities for continuation and expansion. The following are examples of ongoing research programs that reflect the chronology of evidence-based research and best practices in home health.

- *Omaha System* – The Omaha System is one of the twelve classification systems or standardized terminologies recognized by ANA. Four federally funded studies were conducted between 1975 and 1993 to develop and refine the Omaha System and to establish reliability, validity, and usability. Since then, more than 50 unique studies have been conducted by clinicians, managers, educators, students, and researchers; the studies were organized into eight categories and summarized (Martin, 2005; Monsen & Kerr, 2004; Omaha System, 2006). Most have been published in journals, books, or online.

- *Transitional care* – In the 1980s, Brooten and her colleagues compared outcomes and costs when very low birth weight infants remained hospitalized or were cared for at home by advanced practice nurses, and then expanded their studies to include women and elders (Brooten, et al., 2002 & 2003). McCorkle evolved her symptom distress research to include end-of-life and oncology concerns as well as caregivers' psychosocial status (Jepson et al., 1999; Walke et al., 2006). In 1989, Naylor and Bowles began to study high-risk elders and the discharge planning process (Bowles, 2000; Naylor et al., 2005).

- *Visiting Nurse Service (VNS) of New York* – The VNS of New York established a home health research center in 1994. Its sound research and practice improvement initiative has enabled it to attract major grants from private philanthropies and government funding agencies and increasingly to work collaboratively with the home care industry, academic institutions, and quality improvement organizations to improve geriatric care. The center's initiatives focus on three main areas: improving the quality, cost-effectiveness, and outcomes of home health services; analyzing and influencing public policies that affect home-based care; and supporting communities that promote successful aging in place (Feldman et al., 2004 and 2005; McDonald et al., 2005; Murtaugh et al., 2005).

- *Outcome and Assessment Information Set (OASIS)* – OASIS data are used for home health regulation, reimbursement, clinical purposes, and increasingly in research. Studies have examined inter-rater reliability and accuracy of OASIS (Madigan & Fortinsky, 2004; Madigan, Tullai-McGuinness, & Fortinsky, 2003). OASIS data have been used to analyze and evaluate home health clinical outcomes including outcomes for wound healing and home health service use and adverse events among home health patients (Madigan, 2001; Madigan & Tullai-McGuinness, 2004).

- *Work environment* – Through conducting focus groups with home health staff nurses and subsequent analysis, Flynn and Deatrick (2003) identified home care agency attributes important to the support of professional practice and job satisfaction. In a subsequent survey of home health nurses, Flynn (2005) identified the ten traits most important to nurses in supporting professional practice. Flynn and colleagues (2005) pooled survey data from home health nurses with an existing data set of hospital-based nurses to determine whether the core set of organizational traits of the nursing practice environment is similarly valued. The program of research on the work environment is still being extended into home health settings (Flynn, 2007).

- *Telehealth* – This is an emerging area of research that is directly linked to home healthcare clinical practice, policy, and administration. While telehealth vendors conduct product research which is limited in scope, others have developed programs of research that advance the science related to the application of telehealth in the home care setting. Current telehealth studies focus on quality of life, impact on patient outcomes, customer satisfaction, safety, and cost comparisons between home visits and the integrative use of telehealth. Some of the early and continuing studies were conducted by Dansky, Palmer, Shea, and Bowles (2001), Dansky, Bowles, and Palmer (1999), and Bowles and Baugh (2007). Their research has focused on the impact of telehealth intervention on patient outcomes. A group of Minnesota researchers investigated the important relationship of telehealth to patient problems, home health nurse interventions, and patient outcomes (Demiris, Speedie, & Finkelstein, 2000; Finkelstein, Speedie, & Potthoff, 2006).

Summary

Because of demographic changes in the population and technological advances, home health nursing continues to be one of the most rapidly growing and changing specialties. Today home health nurses provide skilled care in the home that was not anticipated a few years ago. Home health nurses must be expert in assessment and clinical decision-making skills that form the foundation for home health nursing practice. These skills, combined with a positive attitude and the willingness and ability to adapt to the ever-changing healthcare environment and technology, will help patients and their families and other caregivers to achieve optimal outcomes.

Given the current pandemic warnings and increasing numbers of reports of natural and man-made disasters, home health nurses will experience additional challenges as the home becomes more often the point of care delivery. Home health nurses will be called upon to coordinate and deliver care unlike ever before. The updated scope of practice statement and revised standards of home health nursing practice are meant to guide, define, and direct home health professional nursing practice today as well as in the future.

APPENDIX A. HOME HEALTH NURSING: SCOPE & STANDARDS OF PRACTICE (2007)

The content in this appendix is not current and is of historical significance only.

STANDARDS OF HOME HEALTH NURSING PRACTICE
STANDARDS OF PRACTICE

STANDARD 1. ASSESSMENT
The home health nurse collects comprehensive data pertinent to the patient's health or the situation.

Measurement Criteria:

The home health nurse:

- Collects physical, psychosocial, and environmental data in a systematic, ongoing process.
- Involves the patient, family, and other healthcare providers in holistic data collection.
- Prioritizes data collection activities based on the patient's immediate condition, or anticipated needs of the patient or situation.
- Uses appropriate evidence-based assessment techniques and instruments in collecting pertinent data.
- Uses analytical tools and critical thinking.
- Synthesizes available data, information, and knowledge relevant to the situation to identify patterns and variances.
- Documents relevant data in a retrievable format.

Additional Measurement Criteria for the Advanced Practice Home Health Nurse:

The advanced practice home health nurse:

- Initiates and interprets diagnostic tests and procedures relevant to the patient's current status.
- Conducts comprehensive and in-depth assessments that identify the patient's specialized needs.

APPENDIX A. HOME HEALTH NURSING: SCOPE & STANDARDS OF PRACTICE (2007)

The content in this appendix is not current and is of historical significance only.

STANDARD 2. DIAGNOSIS
The home health nurse analyzes the assessment data to determine the diagnoses or issues.

Measurement Criteria:

The home health nurse:

- Derives the diagnoses and problems based on assessment data.
- Validates the diagnoses or issues with the patient, family, and other healthcare providers.
- Documents diagnoses or issues in a manner that facilitates the determination of the expected outcomes and plan.

Additional Measurement Criteria for the Advanced Practice Home Health Nurse:

The advanced practice home health nurse:

- Compares and contrasts clinical findings with normal and abnormal variations or developmental events systematically in order to formulate a differential diagnosis.
- Uses complex data and information obtained during interview, examination, and diagnostic procedures in identifying diagnoses.
- Assists staff in developing and maintaining competency in the diagnostic process.

APPENDIX A. HOME HEALTH NURSING: SCOPE & STANDARDS OF PRACTICE (2007)

The content in this appendix is not current and is of historical significance only.

STANDARD 3. OUTCOMES IDENTIFICATION
The home health nurse identifies expected outcomes in a plan individualized to the patient and the situation.

Measurement Criteria:

The home health nurse:

- Collaborates with the patient, family, and other healthcare providers in formulating expected outcomes.
- Derives culturally appropriate expected outcomes from the diagnoses.
- Considers associated risks, benefits, costs, current scientific evidence, and clinical expertise when formulating expected outcomes.
- Defines expected outcomes in terms of the patient, patient values, ethical considerations, environment, or situation with such consideration as associated risks, benefits and costs, and current scientific evidence.
- Individualizes expected outcomes in terms of the patient, patient values, ethical considerations, and the environment.
- Includes a time estimate for attainment of expected outcomes.
- Develops expected outcomes that provide direction for continuity of care.
- Modifies expected outcomes based on changes in the status of the patient or evaluation of the situation.
- Documents expected outcomes as measurable goals.

Additional Measurement Criteria for the Advanced Practice Home Health Nurse:

The advanced practice home health nurse:

- Identifies expected outcomes that incorporate scientific evidence and are achievable through implementation of evidence-based practices.

Continued ▶

APPENDIX A. HOME HEALTH NURSING: SCOPE & STANDARDS OF PRACTICE (2007)

The content in this appendix is not current and is of historical significance only.

- Identifies expected outcomes that incorporate cost and clinical effectiveness, patient satisfaction, and continuity and consistency among providers.
- Uses clinical guidelines that support positive patient outcomes.
- Analyzes the outcome of home health care for specific patient populations to make recommendations for improvement in care delivery systems.

APPENDIX A. HOME HEALTH NURSING: SCOPE & STANDARDS OF PRACTICE (2007)

The content in this appendix is not current and is of historical significance only.

STANDARD 4. PLANNING

The home health nurse develops a plan that prescribes strategies and alternatives to attain expected outcomes.

Measurement Criteria:

The home health nurse:

- Develops an individualized plan considering patient beliefs, values, characteristics and the situation (e.g., age- and culturally appropriate, environmentally sensitive).

- Develops the plan in conjunction with the patient, family and other caregivers, members of the interdisciplinary team, and others.

- Includes strategies within the plan that address each of the identified diagnoses or issues, which may include strategies for promotion and restoration of health and prevention of illness, injury, and disease.

- Provides for continuity within the plan.

- Incorporates an implementation pathway or timeline within the plan.

- Establishes the plan to provide direction to others members of the healthcare team.

- Develops the plan to reflect current statutes, rules and regulations, and standards.

- Integrates current trends and research in the planning process.

- Considers the economic impact of the plan.

- Uses standardized language or recognized terminology to document the plan.

Additional Measurement Criteria for the Advanced Practice Home Health Nurse:

The advanced practice home health nurse:

- Identifies strategies that reflect current evidence, research, literature, and expert clinical knowledge.

- Selects or designs strategies to meet the multifaceted needs of complex patients.

Standard 5. Implementation
The home health nurse implements the individualized patient plan.

(Implementation includes direct care and coordination of care and teaching.)

Measurement Criteria:

The home health nurse:

- Implements the individualized patient plan in a safe and timely manner.
- Uses evidence-based interventions and treatments.
- Uses the plan to provide direction to other members of the healthcare team.
- Documents implementation and changes to the identified plan.

Additional Measurement Criteria for the Advanced Practice Home Health Nurse:

The advanced practice home health nurse:

- Promotes enhanced interdisciplinary and intradisciplinary practice.
- Institutes new evidence-based knowledge and strategies to initiate change in nursing care practices if desired outcomes are not achieved.

APPENDIX A. HOME HEALTH NURSING: SCOPE & STANDARDS OF PRACTICE (2007)

The content in this appendix is not current and is of historical significance only.

STANDARD 5A: COORDINATION OF CARE
The home health nurse coordinates care delivery.

Measurement Criteria:

The home health nurse:

- Coordinates implementation of the plan.
- Facilitates effective uses of resources and systems.
- Uses family, community, financial, and technological resources and systems to implement the plan.
- Collaborates with nursing colleagues and other disciplines to implement the plan.
- Documents the coordination of care.

Measurement Criteria for the Advanced Practice Home Health Nurse:

The advanced practice home health nurse:

- Synthesizes data and information to prescribe necessary system and community support measures, including environmental modifications.
- Provides leadership in the coordination of multidisciplinary healthcare teams for integrated delivery of patient care services.
- Coordinates system and community resources that enhance delivery of care across continuums.

APPENDIX A. HOME HEALTH NURSING: SCOPE & STANDARDS OF PRACTICE (2007)

The content in this appendix is not current and is of historical significance only.

STANDARD 5B: HEALTH TEACHING AND HEALTH PROMOTION

The home health nurse employs strategies to promote health and a safe environment.

Measurement Criteria:

The home health nurse:

- Provides health teaching that addresses such topics as healthy lifestyles, risk-reducing behaviors, home safety, medication management, developmental needs, activities of daily living, and preventive self-care.

- Uses health promotion and health teaching methods appropriate to the situation and the patient's developmental level, learning needs, readiness, ability to learn, language preference, and culture.

- Evaluates the effectiveness of teaching by assessing the patient's learning.

Additional Measurement Criteria for the Advanced Practice Home Health Nurse:

The advanced practice home health nurse:

- Synthesizes empirical evidence on risk behaviors, learning theories, behavioral change theories, motivational theories, epidemiology, and other related theories and frameworks when designing health information and patient education.

- Designs health information and patient education appropriate to the patient's developmental level, learning needs, readiness to learn, and cultural values and beliefs.

- Evaluates health information resources within the area of practice for accuracy, readability, and comprehensibility to help patients access quality health information.

The content in this appendix is not current and is of historical significance only.

STANDARD 5C: CONSULTATION
The advanced practice home health nurse provides consultation to influence the identified plan, enhance the abilities of others, and effect change.

Measurement Criteria for the Advanced Practice Home Health Nurse:

The advanced practice home health nurse:

- Synthesizes clinical data, theoretical frameworks, and evidence when providing consultation.

- Facilitates the effectiveness of a consultation by involving the patient and staff in decision-making and negotiating role responsibilities.

- Provides consultation to facilitate organizational change.

APPENDIX A. HOME HEALTH NURSING: SCOPE & STANDARDS OF PRACTICE (2007)

The content in this appendix is not current and is of historical significance only.

STANDARD 5D: PRESCRIPTIVE AUTHORITY AND TREATMENT

The advanced practice home health nurse uses prescriptive authority, procedures, referrals, treatments, and therapies in accordance with state and federal laws and regulations.

Measurement Criteria for the Advanced Practice Home Health Nurse:

The advanced practice home health nurse:

- Prescribes evidence-based treatments, therapies, and procedures considering the patient's comprehensive healthcare needs.

- Prescribes pharmacologic agents based on a current knowledge of pharmacology and physiology.

- Prescribes specific pharmacological agents and treatments based on clinical indicators, the patient's status and needs, and the results of diagnostic and laboratory tests.

- Evaluates therapeutic and potential adverse effects of pharmacological and non-pharmacological treatments.

- Provides patients with information about intended effects and potential adverse effects of proposed prescriptive therapies.

- Provides information about costs and alternative treatments and procedures, as appropriate.

The content in this appendix is not current and is of historical significance only.

STANDARD 6. EVALUATION
The home health nurse evaluates progress toward attainment of outcomes.

Measurement Criteria:

The home health nurse:

- Conducts a systematic, ongoing evaluation of the patient's outcomes prescribed by the plan and the timeline.
- Includes the patient and others in the evaluative process.
- Evaluates the effectiveness of the planned strategies in relation to patient responses and the attainment of the expected outcomes.
- Uses ongoing assessment data to revise the diagnoses, plan, and implementation strategies as needed to promote optimal patient outcomes.
- Discusses the results with the patient and others involved in the care in accordance with state and federal laws and regulations.
- Documents the results of the evaluation.

Additional Measurement Criteria for the Advanced Practice Home Health Nurse:

The advanced practice home health nurse:

- Evaluates the accuracy of the diagnosis and effectiveness of the interventions in relation to the patient's attainment of expected outcomes.
- Synthesizes the results of the evaluation to determine the impact of the plan on the affected patients, families, groups, communities, and institutions.
- Uses the results of the evaluation to make or recommend process or structural changes including policy, procedure, or protocol documentation.

APPENDIX A. HOME HEALTH NURSING: SCOPE & STANDARDS OF PRACTICE (2007)

The content in this appendix is not current and is of historical significance only.

STANDARDS OF PROFESSIONAL PERFORMANCE

STANDARD 7. QUALITY OF PRACTICE
The home health nurse systematically enhances the quality and effectiveness of nursing practice.

Measurement Criteria:

The home health nurse:

- Demonstrates quality through the application of the nursing process in a responsible, accountable, and ethical manner.
- Uses the results of quality improvement activities to initiate changes in nursing practice and in the healthcare delivery system.
- Incorporates creativity and innovation in nursing practice to improve the quality of care delivery.
- Incorporates evidence-based knowledge into nursing practice to enhance patient outcomes.
- Participates in quality improvement activities. Such activities may include:
  - Identifying aspects of practice important for quality monitoring.
  - Using indicators developed to monitor quality and effectiveness of nursing practice.
  - Collecting data to monitor quality and effectiveness of nursing practice.
  - Analyzing quality indicators and other data to identify opportunities for improving nursing practice and patient outcomes.
  - Formulating recommendations based on quality indicators and other data to improve nursing practice and patient outcomes.
  - Implementing activities based on quality indicators and other data to improve nursing practice and patient outcomes.
  - Analyzing, evaluating, and recommending new technologies to improve patient outcomes.

Continued ▶

APPENDIX A. HOME HEALTH NURSING: SCOPE & STANDARDS OF PRACTICE (2007)

The content in this appendix is not current and is of historical significance only.

- Developing, implementing, and evaluating policies, procedures, and guidelines to improve the quality of nursing practice and patient outcomes.
- Serving as the interdisciplinary team leader or member to evaluate clinical care and health services.
- Determining cost-effective care based on patient need.
- Analyzing factors related to safety, satisfaction, effectiveness, and cost–benefit options.
- Identifying barriers within organizations.

Additional Measurement Criteria for the Advanced Practice Home Health Nurse:

The advanced practice home health nurse:

- Obtains and maintains professional certification if it is available in the area of expertise.
- Designs quality improvement initiatives.
- Implements initiatives to evaluate the need for change.
- Evaluates the practice environment and quality of nursing care rendered in relation to existing evidence, identifying opportunities for the initiation, support, and use of research.
- Analyzes barriers within organizations.
- Implements processes to remove or decrease barriers within organizations.

Standard 8. Education
The home health nurse attains knowledge and competency that reflects current nursing practice.

Measurement Criteria:

The home health nurse:

- Identifies learning needs through self-reflection and inquiry.
- Participates in ongoing educational activities related to appropriate knowledge bases and professional issues.
- Demonstrates a commitment to lifelong learning.
- Seeks experiences that reflect current practice in order to maintain skills and competence in clinical practice or role performance.
- Acquires knowledge and skills appropriate to the specialty area, practice setting, role, or situation.
- Maintains competencies that include interpersonal, technical, and information technology skills.
- Maintains professional records that provide evidence of competency and lifelong learning.
- Seeks experiences and formal and independent learning activities to maintain and develop clinical and professional skills and knowledge.

Additional Measurement Criteria for the Advanced Practice Home Health Nurse:

The advanced practice home health nurse:

- Uses current healthcare research findings and other evidence to expand clinical knowledge, enhance role performance, and increase knowledge of professional issues.

APPENDIX A. HOME HEALTH NURSING: SCOPE & STANDARDS OF PRACTICE (2007)

The content in this appendix is not current and is of historical significance only.

STANDARD 9. PROFESSIONAL PRACTICE EVALUATION

The home health nurse evaluates one's own nursing practice in relation to professional practice standards and guidelines, relevant statutes, rules, and regulations.

Measurement Criteria:

The home health nurse's practice reflects the application of knowledge of current practice standards, guidelines, statutes, rules, and regulations.

The home health nurse:

- Provides age-appropriate care in a culturally and linguistically sensitive manner.
- Engages in self-evaluation of practice on a regular basis, identifying areas of strength as well as areas in which professional development would be beneficial.
- Incorporates feedback from patients, peers, and professional colleagues into professional practice development.
- Participates in systematic peer review as appropriate.
- Takes action to achieve goals identified during the evaluation process.
- Provides rationales for practice beliefs, decisions, and actions as part of the informal and formal evaluation processes.

Additional Measurement Criteria for the Advanced Practice Home Health Nurse:

The advanced practice home health nurse:

- Engages in a formal process seeking feedback regarding one's own practice from patients, peers, professional colleagues, and others.
- Analyzes one's practice in relation to advanced certification requirements.

APPENDIX A. HOME HEALTH NURSING: SCOPE & STANDARDS OF PRACTICE (2007)

The content in this appendix is not current and is of historical significance only.

STANDARD 10. COLLEGIALITY
The home health nurse interacts with peers and colleagues, and contributes to their professional development.

Measurement Criteria:

The home health nurse:

- Shares knowledge and skills with peers and colleagues as evidenced by such activities as patient care conferences or presentations at formal or informal meetings.
- Provides peers and colleagues with feedback regarding their practice or role performance.
- Interacts with peers and colleagues to enhance one's own professional nursing practice or role performance.
- Maintains a supportive relationship with peers and colleagues that increases the effectiveness of the team.
- Contributes to an environment that is conducive to the education of healthcare professionals.
- Contributes to a supportive and healthy work environment.
- Mentors others in home health.

Additional Measurement Criteria for the Advanced Practice Home Health Nurse:

The advanced practice home health nurse:

- Models expert practice to interdisciplinary team members and healthcare consumers.
- Participates in interdisciplinary teams that contribute to role development and advanced nursing practice and health care.

APPENDIX A. HOME HEALTH NURSING: SCOPE & STANDARDS OF PRACTICE (2007)

The content in this appendix is not current and is of historical significance only.

STANDARD 11. COLLABORATION
The home health nurse collaborates with the patient, family, and others in the conduct of nursing practice.

Measurement Criteria:

The home health nurse:

- Communicates with the patient, family, and healthcare providers regarding patient care and the nurse's role in providing that care.

- Collaborates in creating a documented plan focused on outcomes and decisions related to care and delivery of services that indicates communication with patients, families, and others.

- Partners with others to effect change and generate positive outcomes through knowledge of the patient or situation.

- Documents referrals, including provisions for continuity of care.

Additional Measurement Criteria for the Advanced Practice Home Health Nurse:

The advanced practice home health nurse:

- Partners with other disciplines to enhance patient care through interdisciplinary activities and opportunities in education, consultation, management, technological development, or research.

- Facilitates an interdisciplinary process with other members of the healthcare team.

- Documents plan-of-care communications, rationales for plan-of-care changes, and collaborative discussions to improve patient care.

STANDARD 12. ETHICS
The home health nurse integrates ethical principles into all areas of practice.

Measurement Criteria:

The home health nurse:

- Uses *Code of Ethics for Nurses with Interpretive Statements* (ANA, 2001) to guide practice.
- Delivers care in a manner that preserves and protects patient autonomy, dignity, and rights.
- Maintains patient confidentiality within legal and regulatory parameters.
- Serves as a patient advocate assisting patients in developing skills for self advocacy.
- Maintains a therapeutic and professional patient–nurse relationship within appropriate professional role boundaries.
- Contributes to resolving ethical issues of patients, colleagues, or systems as evidenced in such activities as participating on ethics committees.
- Reports illegal, incompetent, or impaired practices.
- Informs the patient of the risks, benefits, and outcomes of healthcare regimens.
- Participates in interdisciplinary teams that address ethical risks, benefits, and outcomes.
- Maintains one's own health and well-being through health-promoting behaviors.

Additional Measurement Criteria for the Advanced Practice Home Health Nurse:

The advanced practice home health nurse:

- Analyzes ethical issues within organizations.
- Participates in interdisciplinary teams that address ethical risks, benefits, and outcomes.

APPENDIX A. HOME HEALTH NURSING: SCOPE & STANDARDS OF PRACTICE (2007)

The content in this appendix is not current and is of historical significance only.

STANDARD 13. RESEARCH
The home health nurse integrates research findings into practice.

Measurement Criteria:

The home health nurse:

- Uses the best available evidence, including research findings, to guide practice decisions.

- Actively participates in research activities at various levels appropriate to the nurse's level of education and position. Such activities may include:

  - Identifying clinical problems specific to nursing research (patient care and nursing practice).

  - Participating in data collection (surveys, pilot projects, formal studies).

  - Participating in a formal committee or program.

  - Sharing research activities and findings with colleagues and others.

  - Conducting research.

  - Using research findings in the development of policies, procedures, and standards of practice in patient care.

  - Incorporating research as a basis for learning.

Additional Measurement Criteria for the Advanced Practice Home Health Nurse:

The advanced practice home health nurse:

- Contributes to nursing knowledge by conducting or synthesizing research that discovers, examines, and evaluates knowledge, theories, criteria, and creative approaches to improve home health practice.

- Formally disseminates research findings through activities such as presentations, publications, consultation, and journal clubs.

- Critically analyzes and interprets research for application to practice.

- Develops evidence-based education programs to improve and standardize the delivery of evidence-based care for the nursing team.

APPENDIX A. HOME HEALTH NURSING: SCOPE & STANDARDS OF PRACTICE (2007)

The content in this appendix is not current and is of historical significance only.

STANDARD 14. RESOURCE UTILIZATION

The home health nurse considers factors related to safety, effectiveness, cost, and impact on practice in the planning and delivery of nursing services.

Measurement Criteria:

The home health nurse:

- Evaluates factors such as safety, effectiveness, availability, cost and benefits, efficiencies, and impact on practice when choosing practice options that would result in the same expected outcome.

- Assists the patient and family in identifying and securing appropriate and available services to address health-related needs.

- Assigns or delegates tasks, based on the needs and condition of the patient, potential for harm, stability of the patient's condition, complexity of the task, and predictability of the outcome.

- Assists the patient and family in becoming informed consumers about the options, costs, risks, and benefits of treatment and care.

- Uses organizational and community resources to formulate interdisciplinary plans of care.

Additional Measurement Criteria for the Advanced Practice Home Health Nurse:

The advanced practice home health nurse:

- Develops innovative solutions for patient care problems that address effective resource utilization and maintenance of quality.

- Develops evaluation strategies to demonstrate cost effectiveness, cost–benefit, and efficiency factors associated with nursing practice.

- Analyzes the outcomes of care related to organizational care delivery for the populations served to make recommendations for improvement in care delivery systems of home healthcare patients.

STANDARD 15. LEADERSHIP
The home health nurse provides leadership in the professional practice setting and the profession.

Measurement Criteria:

The home health nurse:

- Engages in team efforts as a team leader, team builder, and team player.
- Works to create and maintain healthy work environments in local, regional, national, or international communities.
- Displays the ability to define a clear vision, the associated goals, and a plan to implement and measure progress.
- Demonstrates a commitment to lifelong learning for self and others.
- Teaches others to succeed, by mentoring and other supportive strategies.
- Exhibits creativity and flexibility through times of change.
- Demonstrates energy, excitement, and a passion for quality work.
- Willingly accepts mistakes by self and others, thereby creating a culture in which risk-taking is not only safe, but expected.
- Inspires loyalty by valuing people as the most precious asset in an organization.
- Directs the coordination of care across settings and among caregivers, including oversight of licensed and unlicensed personnel in any assigned or delegated tasks.
- Serves in key roles in the work setting by participating in committees, councils, and administrative teams.
- Promotes advancement of the profession through participation in professional organizations.
- Advocates in the political arena for healthcare systems that eliminate health disparities and promote excellent health outcomes for all members of society.

Additional Measurement Criteria for the Advanced Practice Home Health Nurse:

The advanced practice home health nurse:

- Works to influence decision-making bodies to improve patient care.
- Provides direction to enhance the effectiveness of the healthcare team.
- Initiates and revises protocols or guidelines to reflect evidence-based practice, to reflect accepted changes in care management, or to address emerging problems.
- Promotes communication of information and advancement of the profession through writing, publishing, and presentations for professional or lay audiences.
- Designs innovations to effect change in practice and improve health outcomes.

APPENDIX A. HOME HEALTH NURSING: SCOPE & STANDARDS OF PRACTICE (2007)

The content in this appendix is not current and is of historical significance only.

Glossary

Advocacy. Actions intended to maximize patient autonomy and self-determinism through informing, supporting, and affirming a patient's decisions.

Agency/Organization. A formal entity that runs the home care department and that provides home health services to patients of a home health agency or hospital.

Assessment. A systematic, dynamic process by which the registered nurse, through interaction with the patient, significant others, and healthcare practitioners, collects and analyzes data about the patient. Data may include the following dimensions: physical, psychological, socio-cultural, spiritual, cognitive, functional abilities, developmental, economic, and lifestyle.

Care management. An organized system or process for delivering health care to a patient, including assessment, development of a plan of care, initiation and coordination of referrals and services, and evaluation of care. As a care manager, the home health nurse focuses on meeting the comprehensive needs of patients while maximizing appropriate resources and service utilization and acting as a patient advocate.

Caregiver. Anyone who provides care to a patient.

Clinical practice guidelines. Systematic statements designed to help clinicians in making decisions about care. Generally, a group of expert decision-makers are convened to perform a systematic literature review and make specific recommendations based on the evidence.

Complementary and Alternative Medicine (CAM). A group of diverse medical and healthcare systems, practices, and products not presently considered as part of conventional or D.O. (doctor of osteopathy) degrees and by physical therapists, psychologists, and registered nurses. Some healthcare providers practice both CAM and conventional medicine. *Complementary medicine* is used *together with* conventional medicine (e.g., aromatherapy to help lessen a patient's discomfort following surgery). *Alternative medicine* is used *in place of* conventional medicine (e.g., a special diet to treat cancer instead of undergoing surgery, radiation, or chemotherapy).

Cultural therapy. Therapies and treatments used by ethnic, religious, or other cultural groups to promote health and healing. These therapies are usually neither helpful nor harmful from a professional perspective.

Diagnosis. A clinical judgment about the patient's response to actual or potential health conditions or needs. Diagnoses provide the basis for determination of a plan of care to achieve expected outcomes. Registered nurses use nursing or medical diagnoses depending on educational and clinical preparation and legal authority.

Disease management. Coordinated healthcare interventions aimed at specific populations with conditions in which patient self-care efforts are significant, such as heart failure, diabetes, and chronic lung disease.

Electronic health record (EHR). Longitudinal collection of clinical and demographic patient-specific information, stored in a computer-readable format.

Evaluation. The process of determining the progress toward attainment of expected outcomes. Outcomes include the effectiveness of care when addressing one's practice.

Evidence-based practice. A process founded on the collection, interpretation, and integration of valid, important, and applicable patient-reported, clinician-observed, or research-derived evidence. The best available evidence, moderated by patient circumstances and preferences, is applied to improve the quality of clinical judgments.

Family. Family of origin or significant others as identified by the patient.

Home. The patient's residence, which may include a private home or an assisted living or personal care facility.

Home health nursing. A specialized area of nursing practice, rooted in community health nursing, that delivers care in the residence of the patient.

Implementation. Activities such as teaching, monitoring, providing, counseling, delegating, and coordinating.

Information management. Integration of clinical, demographic, financial, administrative, and staffing data; manipulation or processing of these data; and production of various reports that transform data into meaningful information for decision-making.

APPENDIX A. HOME HEALTH NURSING: SCOPE & STANDARDS OF PRACTICE (2007)

The content in this appendix is not current and is of historical significance only.

Interdisciplinary team. A team that includes members from different professions and occupations who work together closely and communicate frequently to optimize care for the patient. Each team member contributes knowledge, skills, and experience to support and augment the contributions of other team members.

Outcomes. Measurable changes in a patient's health status between two or more points in time; in particular, the intervention, intermediate, and end points of nursing and health care.

Plan of care. Comprehensive outline of care to be delivered to attain expected outcomes. It can include prescriptive plans of all disciplines involved with the patient's home health care.

Qualitative data. Pertinent subjective patient-specific narrative details that are derived from interviews, documents, and observation of interactions; the data collector focuses on the whole to give meaning to life experiences.

Quantitative data. Pertinent objective patient-specific numerical details that can be counted and measured consistently; the data collector focuses on the parts to identify positive or negative trends.

Self-management. A patient, family, or caregiver managing an illness or disability independently, keeping the patient as healthy as possible on a daily basis, and identifying early signs of trouble that need additional medical or nursing intervention.

Standard. An authoritative statement defined and promoted by the profession, by which the quality of practice, service, or education can be evaluated.

Standards of care. Authoritative statements that describe a competent level of clinical nursing practice demonstrated through assessment, diagnosis, outcomes identification, planning, implementation, and evaluation.

Standards of nursing practice. Authoritative statements that describe a level of care or performance common to the profession of nursing, by which the quality of nursing practice can be judged. Standards of clinical nursing practice include both standards of care and standards of professional performance.

The content in this appendix is not current and is of historical significance only.

Standards of professional performance. Authoritative statements that describe a competent level of behavior in the professional role, including quality of practice, education, professional performance evaluation, collegiality, collaboration, ethics, research, resource utilization, and leadership.

APPENDIX A. HOME HEALTH NURSING: SCOPE & STANDARDS OF PRACTICE (2007)

The content in this appendix is not current and is of historical significance only.

REFERENCES

American Nurses Association (ANA). (1999). *Scope and standards of home health nursing practice.* Washington, DC: American Nurses Publishing.

———. (2001). *Code of ethics for nurses with interpretive statements.* Washington, DC: American Nurses Publishing.

———. (2003) *Nursing's social policy statement* (2nd ed.). Washington, DC: Nursesbooks.org.

———. (2004) *Nursing: Scope and standards of practice.* Washington, DC: Nursesbooks.org.

———. (2005) *Recognition of a specialty, approval of scope statements, and acknowledgment of nursing practice standards.* Washington, DC: Nursesbooks.org.

———. (2006). *ANA recognized terminologies and data element sets.* Retrieved September 25, 2007, from http://nursingworld.org/npii/.

Bowles, K.H. (2000). Patient problems and nurse interventions during acute care and discharge planning. *Journal of Cardiovascular Nursing, 14*(3), 29–41.

Bowles, K.H., & Baugh, A.C. (2007). Applying research evidence to optimize telehomecare. *Journal of Cardiovascular Nursing, 22*(1), 5–15.

Brantley, D., Laney-Cummings, K., & Spivack, R. (2004). *Innovation, demand, and investment in telehealth.* U.S. Dept. of Commerce: Office of Technology Policy. Retrieved September 25, 2007 from http://www.technology.gov.reports/TechPolicy/Telehealth/2004Report.pdf.

Brooten, D., Naylor, M.D., York, R., Brown, L.P., Hazard, Munro B., et al. (2002). Lessons learned from testing the quality cost model of advanced practice nursing (APN) transitional care. *Journal of Nursing Scholarship, 34*(4), 369–375.

APPENDIX A. HOME HEALTH NURSING: SCOPE & STANDARDS OF PRACTICE (2007)

The content in this appendix is not current and is of historical significance only.

Brooten, D., Youngblut, J.M., Deatrick, J., Naylor, M., & York, R. (2003). Patient problems, advanced practice nursing (APN) interventions, time and contacts across five patient groups. *Journal of Nursing Scholarship*, 35(1), 73–79.

Centers for Disease Control and Prevention (CDC). (2004). *The burden of chronic diseases and their risk factors: National and state perspectives 2004*. CDC. Retrieved September 25, 2007, from http://www.cdc.gov/nccdphp/burdenbook2004/index.htm.

Clark, J., & Lang, N.M. (1992). Nursing's next advance: An international classification for nursing practice. *International Nursing Review*, 39(4), 109–111, 128.

Dansky, K.H., Bowles, K.H., & Palmer, L. (1999). How telehomecare affects patients. *Caring, XVIII*(8), 10–14.

Dansky, K.H., Palmer, L., Shea, D., & Bowles, K.H. (2001). Cost analysis of telehomecare. *Telemedicine and e-Health*, 7(3), 225–232.

Demiris, G., Speedie, S., & Finkelstein, S. (2000). A questionnaire for the assessment of patients' impressions of the risks and benefits of home telecare. *Telemedicine and e-Health*, 6(5), 278–284.

Feldman, P.H., Murtaugh, C.M., Pezzin, L.E., McDonald, M.V., & Peng, T.R. (2005). Just-in-time evidence-based email "reminders" in home health care: Impact on patient outcomes. *Health Services Research*, 40(3), 849–864.

Feldman, P.H., Peng, T.R., Murtaugh, C.M., Kelleher, C., Donelson, S.M., McCann, M.E., et al. (2004). A randomized intervention to improve heart failure outcomes in community-based home care. *Home Health Care Services Quarterly*, 23(1), 1–23.

Finkelstein, S.M., Speedie, S.M., & Potthoff, S. (2006). Home telehealth improves clinical outcomes at lower cost for home healthcare. *Telemedicine and e-Health*, 12(2), 128–136.

The content in this appendix is not current and is of historical significance only.

Flynn, L. (2005). The importance of work environment: Evidence-based strategies for enhancing nurse retention. *Home Healthcare Nurse, 23*(6), 366–371.

Flynn, L. (2007). Extending work environment research into home health settings. *Western Journal of Nursing Research, 29*, 200–212.

Flynn, L., Carryer, J., & Budge, C. (2005). Organizational attributes valued by hospital, home care, and district nurses in the United States and New Zealand. *Journal of Nursing Scholarship, 37*(1), 67–72.

Flynn, L., & Deatrick, J.A. (2003). Home care nurses' descriptions of important agency attributes. *Journal of Nursing Scholarship, 35*(4), 385–390.

Harris, M. (2006). We need your input…This is your opportunity to have a voice in the future of your profession. *Home Healthcare Nurse, 24*(3), 133–135.

Humphrey, C.J., & Milone-Nuzzo, P. (1996–1999). *Manual of home care nursing orientation*. Gaithersburg: Aspen.

Humphrey, C.J., & Milone-Nuzzo, P. (2008). *Manual of home care nursing orientation*. Louisville, KY: C.J. Humphrey Associates.

Huston, C.J. (2006). *Professional issues in nursing: Challenges and opportunities*. Philadelphia: Lippincott Williams and Wilkins, pp. 85–98, 256–261.

Jepson, C., McCorkle, R., Adler, D., Nuamah, I., & Lusk, E. (1999). Effects of home care on caregivers' psychological status. *Image: Journal of Nursing Scholarship, 31*(2), 115–120.

Joint Commission International Center for Patient Safety. *2007 National patient safety goals: Home care.* Retrieved September 25, 2007 from http://www.jcipatientsafety.org.

Madigan, E.A. (2001). Comparison of home health care outcomes and service use for patients with wound/skin diagnoses. *Outcomes Management for Nursing Practice, 5*(2), 63–67.

APPENDIX A. HOME HEALTH NURSING: SCOPE & STANDARDS OF PRACTICE (2007)

The content in this appendix is not current and is of historical significance only.

Madigan, E.A., & Fortinsky, R.H. (2004). Inter-rater reliability of the outcomes and assessment information set: Results from the field. *Gerontologist, 44*(5), 689–92.

Madigan, E.A., & Tullai-McGuiness, S. (2004). An examination of the most frequent adverse events in home care agencies. *Home Healthcare Nurse, 22*(4), 256–62.

Madigan, E.A., Tullai-McGuiness, S., & Fortinsky, R.H. (2003). Accuracy in the outcomes and assessment information set (OASIS): Results of a video simulation. *Research in Nursing and Health, 26*(4), 273–283.

Madigan, E.A., & Vanderboom, C. (2005). Home health nursing research priorities. *Applied Nursing Research, 18*(4), 221–225.

Martin, K.S. (2005). *The Omaha System: A key to practice, documentation, and information management* (2nd ed.). St. Louis: Elsevier.

McDonald, M.V., Pezzin, L.E., Feldman, P.H., Murtaugh, C.M., & Peng, T.R. (2005). Can just-in-time evidence-based "reminders" improve pain management among home health care nurses and their patients? *Journal of Pain and Symptom Management, 29*(5), 474–488.

Mebus, K, & Piskor, B. (2005). Participating in the political process. In M. Harris (Ed.), *Handbook of home health care administration* (4th ed.). Sudbury: Jones and Bartlett.

Monsen, K.A., & Kerr, M.J. (2004). Mining quality documentation for golden outcomes. *Home Health Management and Practice, 16*(3), 192–199.

Murtaugh, C.M., Pezzin, L.E., McDonald, M.V., Feldman, P.H., & Peng, T.R. (2005). Just-in-time evidence-based email "reminders" in home health care: Impact on nurse practices. *Health Services Research, 40*(3), 849–864.

National Association for Home Care & Hospice (NAHC). (2004). *Basic statistics about home care.* Washington, DC; NAHC.

National Association for Home Care & Hospice (NAHC). (2006). *Briggs national quality improvement/hospitalization reduction study.* January

2006. Retrieved September 25, 2007 from http://www.nahc.org/NAHC/CaringComm/eNAHCReport/datacharts/hospredstudy.pdf.

National Association of Clinical Nurse Specialists (NACNS). (2004). *Statement on clinical nurse specialist practice and education*. Harrisburg, PA: NACNS.

Naylor, M.D., Stephens, C., Bowles, K.H., & Bixby, M.B. (2005). Cognitively impaired older adults: From hospital to home. *American Journal of Nursing, 105*(2), 52–61.

Omaha System. (2006). *Overview*. Retrieved September 25, 2007 from http://www.omahasystem.org.

Rogers, E.M. (1995). *Diffusion of innovation* (4th ed.). New York: The Free Press.

Schumacher, K.L. & Marren, J. (2004). Home care nursing for older adults: State of the science. *Nursing Clinics of North America. 39*(3), 443–471.

Stoker, J. (2003). Home care LPN utilization. *Home Healthcare Nurse, 21*(2), 85–89.

U.S. Department of Health and Human Services. (2002). *2001 Report to Congress on telemedicine*. Retrieved September 25, 2007 from http://www.hrsa.gov/telehealth/pubs/report2001.htm.

U.S. Department of Labor, Bureau of Labor Statistics (2006–2007). Occupational Handbook, 2006–07 ed. *Registered Nurses*. Retrieved September 25, 2007 from http://www.bls.gov/oco/ocos083.htm#conditions.

Utterback, K. & Waldo, B. (2005). Matching point of care devices for positive outcomes. *Home Healthcare Nurse, 23*(7), 452–459.

Walke, L.M., Byers, A.L., McCorkle, R., & Fried, T.R. (2006). Symptom assessment in community-dwelling older adults with advanced chronic disease. *Journal of Pain Symptom Management, 31*(1), 31–37.

Wilson, A. (2005). Benchmarking and home health care. In M. Harris (Ed.), *Handbook of home health care administration* (4th ed.) Sudbury: Jones and Bartlett.

World Health Organization (WHO). (2003). *Adherence to long term therapies: Evidence for action*. Retrieved September 25, 2007, from http://www.who.int/chp/knowledge/publications/adherence_report/en/index.html

———. (2007). *International Statistical Classification of Diseases and Related Health Problems, 10th Revision*. Retrieved September 25, 2007, from http://www.who.int/classifications/icd/en/.

The content in this appendix is not current and is of historical significance only.

Bibliography

American Nurses Association (ANA). (1999). *Competencies for telehealth technologies in nursing.* Washington, DC: American Nurses Publishing.

American Nurses Association. (2004). *Nurse administrators: Scope and standards of nursing practice.* Washington, DC: Nursesbooks.org.

Buhler-Wilkerson, K. (2001). *No place like home: A history of nursing and home care in the United States.* Baltimore: Johns Hopkins University Press.

Centers for Medicare & Medicaid Services. (2006). *CMS programs and information.* Retrieved September 25, 2007 from http://www.cms.hhs.gov/.

Cherney, E. (2006). New ways to monitor patients at home, as insurers increasingly cover "telemedicine," companies launch way of devices. *The Wall Street Journal,* April 18, p. D1.

Cimino, J.J. (1998). Desiderata for controlled medical vocabularies in the twenty-first century. *Methods of Information in Medicine, 37*(4–5), 394–403.

Dolan, J., Fitzpatrick, M., & Herrmann, E. (1983). *Nursing in society: A historical perspective* (15th ed.). Philadelphia: Saunders.

Dombi, W.A. (Ed.). (2000). *Home care and hospice law: A handbook for executives.* Washington, DC: Caring Publications.

Donahue, M.P. (1996). *Nursing: The finest art* (2nd ed.). St. Louis: Mosby.

Fesler-Brich, D. (2005). Critical thinking and patient outcomes: A review. *Nursing Outlook, 53*(2), 59–65.

Hegyvary, S.T. (2006). A call for papers on evidence-based problems. *Journal of Nursing Scholarship, 38*(1), 1–2.

Kalisch, P.A., & Kalisch, B.J. (1995). *The advance of American nursing* (3rd ed.). Philadelphia: Lippincott.

Lang, N.M. (Ed.). (1995). *Nursing data systems: The emerging framework.* Washington, DC: American Nurses Publishing.

Milone-Nuzzo, P. (2000). Advanced practice nurses in home care are essential. *Home Healthcare Nurse 18*(1), 22–23.

Milone-Nuzzo, P. (2003). Clinical nurse specialists in home care. *Clinical Nurse Specialist, 17*(5), 234–235.

Neal, J.N., & Madigan, E.A. (2001). *Core curriculum for home health care nursing.* Washington, DC: Home Care University, Home Healthcare Nurses Association.

Robert Wood Johnson Foundation. (2002). *Advanced practice nursing: Pioneering practices in palliative care.* Retrieved September 25, 2007 from http://www.promotingexcellence.org/i4a/pages/Index.cfm?pageID=3775.

Schoesslet, M., & Waldo, M. (2006). The first 18 months in practice: A developmental transition model for the newly graduated nurse. *Journal for Nurses in Staff Development, 22*(2), 47–52.

Stoker, J. (2003). Home care LPN utilization. *Home Healthcare Nurse, 21*(2), 85–89.

Stoker, J., & Phillips, B. (2005). Effective support for certain patient populations: One agency's experience. *Home Healthcare Nurse, 23*(11), 696–698.

Struk, C., Peters, D., & Saba, V. (2006). Community health applications. In V. Saba & K.A. McCormick (Eds.), *Essentials of nursing informatics* (pp. 355–382). New York: McGraw Hill Publishing.

Transforming Clinical Data into Critical Outcome Information: How to Survive in the New Data-driven World. (2004). *Home Health Care Management and Practice, 16*(3), special issue.

U.S. Department of Health and Human Services. (2002). HRSA. Bureau of Health Professions. Division of Nursing. *Nurse practitioner primary care competencies in specialty areas: Adult, family, gerontological, pediatric, and women's health.* Retrieved September 25, 2007, from http://www.nonpf.org/finalaug2002.pdf.

Index

Note: Entries with [2007] indicate an entry from *Home Health Nursing: Scope and Standards of Practice* (2007), reproduced in Appendix A. That information is not current but included for historical value only.

A

Abilities in home health nursing practice, 12, 14, 16, 23, 25, 26, 41, 54, 100, 109, 120, 141. *See also* Knowledge, skills, abilities, and judgment

Access in home health nursing practice, 39

Accountability in home health nursing practice, 5, 21, 28–29, 69, 91

Accountable care organizations (ACOs), 24, 38

ACOs. *See* Accountable care organizations (ACOs)

Activities of daily living (ADLs), 8

ADLs. *See* Activities of daily living (ADLs)

Administrator roles in home health nursing practice, 18–22

Advanced practice registered nurses (APRNs) in home health nursing practice, x, 13, 101
  assessment competencies, 45
  collaboration competencies, 70–71
  consultation competencies, 56
  coordination of care competencies, 53
  diagnosis competencies, 46
  education competencies, 63
  environmental health competencies, 75–76
  ethics competencies, 61
  evaluation competencies, 58–59
  evidence-based practice and research competencies, 64
  health teaching and health promotion competencies, 54–55
  implementation competencies, 52
  leadership competencies, 69
  outcomes identification competencies, 47–48
  planning competencies, 50
  prescriptive authority and treatment competencies, 57
  professional practice evaluation competencies, 72
  quality of practice competencies, 66
  resource utilization competencies, 74

Advocacy in home health nursing practice, 17, 21–22, 28

Affordable Care Act, Patient Protection and, 3–4, 39–40

INDEX

Agencies in home health nursing practice, 2–3, 14, 17, 19, 21, 22, 31
  competencies involving, 49, 61, 68, 69, 71, 74
  financial issues, 38, 39–40
  health care reform and, 39–40
  informatics and telehealth and, 35–36, 37–38
  research and, 31–32
  technology innovation and, 35, 36, 40
  trends and issues of, 24–26
American Nurses Association (ANA), viii, ix, 2, 3, 30, 33, 91, 92, 93, 94, 113, 118
American Nurses Credentialing Center (ANCC), 11
  Magnet Recognition Program, 24
  Pathway to Excellence Program, 24
ANA. *See* American Nurses Association (ANA)
Analysis in home health nursing practice. *See* Critical thinking
ANCC. *See* American Nurses Credentialing Center (ANCC)
APRNs. *See* Advanced practice registered nurses (APRNs)
Assessment in home health nursing practice, 7–8, 96–97
  assessment data, 8, 31, 44, 45, 46, 58, 97, 122, 131
  competencies involving, 44–45
  Standard of Practice, 44–45
  [2007], 121
Attitudes in home health nursing practice, 24, 41, 44, 120
Awareness in home health nursing practice, 30

B

Benefits and costs. *See* Cost and economic controls
Breckinridge, Mary, 1
Budgetary issues. *See* Cost and economic controls

C

Care coordination, 4, 6, 8, 38, 41, 77
  defined, 77. *See also* Coordination of care
Care delivery. *See* Coordination of care
Care management, 10, 12, 14, 15
  defined, 77
Care manager role in home health nursing practice, 10, 12, 15–16
Care plans. *See* Plan of care (POC); Planning
Care recipients. *See* Healthcare consumers
Caregivers, defined, 77
Case management. *See* Care management
Centers for Medicare & Medicaid Services (CMS), 2, 3
Certification and credentialing in home health nursing practice, 11, 13, 19, 66, 99, 133
Characteristics, of home health nursing, 6–7
Clients. *See* Healthcare consumers
Clinical Care Classification, 38
Clinical educator in home health nursing practice, 20–22
Clinical manager in home health nursing practice, 19–20
Clinical nurse specialist (CNS) in home health nursing practice, 13–14, 101–102
  roles, 14
Clinical roles in home health nursing practice, 15–17
Clinical settings in home health nursing practice. *See* Practice environments and settings
CMS. *See* Centers for Medicare & Medicaid Services (CMS)
CNS. *See* Clinical nurse specialist (CNS)
Code of Ethics for Nurses with Interpretive Statements, ix, 27, 91

156 *Home Health Nursing: Scope and Standards of Practice, 2nd Edition*

Collaboration in home health nursing
  practice, 6, 13, 16, 30. *See also*
  Communication
  competencies involving, 70–71
  Standard of Professional
    Performance, 70–71
  [2007], 137
Collegiality in home health nursing
  practice
  Standard of Professional Performance
  [2007], 136
Commitment in home health nursing
  practice, 27–28
Communication in home health nursing
  practice. *See also* Collaboration
  competencies involving, 67
  Standard of Professional
    Performance, 67
Community-based care, 1, 4, 93. *See also*
  Home health nursing practice
Compassion in home health nursing
  practice, 23, 27
Competencies in home health nursing
  practice
  for APRNs, 45, 46, 47–48, 50, 52, 53,
    54–55, 56, 57, 58–59, 61, 63, 64,
    66, 69, 70–71, 72, 74, 75–76
  assessment, 44–45
  collaboration, 70–71
  communication, 67
  consultation, 56
  coordination of care, 53
  diagnosis, 46
  education, 62–63
  environmental health, 75–76
  ethics, 60–61
  evaluation, 58–59
  evidence-based practice and
    research, 64
  for graduate-level prepared home
    health nurse, 45, 46, 47–48, 50,
    52, 53, 54–55, 56, 57, 58–59, 61,
    63, 64, 66, 69, 70–71, 72, 74,
    75–76
  health teaching and health
    promotion, 54–55

implementation, 51–52
leadership, 68–69
outcomes identification, 47–48
planning, 49–50
prescriptive authority and
  treatment, 57
professional practice evaluation, 72
quality of practice, 65–66
resource utilization, 73–74
for RNs, 44–45, 46, 47, 49–50, 51–52,
  53, 54, 58, 60–61, 62, 64, 65–66,
  67, 68–69, 70, 72, 73, 75
Confidentiality and privacy in home
  health nursing practice, 28, 45, 60
Consultation in home health nursing
  practice
  competencies involving, 56
  Standard of Practice, 56
  [2007], 129
Continuity of care, defined, 77
Coordination of care in home health
  nursing practice
  competencies involving, 53
  Standard of Practice, 53
  [2007], 127. *See also* Care
    coordination
Cost and economic controls in home
  health nursing practice, 3, 4, 7, 39–40
Counseling in home health nursing
  practice, 6, 7, 9, 55, 67
Credentialing. *See* Certification and
  credentialing
Criteria in home health nursing
  practice, [2007]
  assessment, 121
  collaboration, 137
  collegiality, 136
  consultation, 129
  coordination of care, 127
  diagnosis, 122
  education, 134
  ethics, 138
  evaluation, 131
  health teaching and health
    promotion, 128

Home Health Nursing: Scope and Standards of Practice, 2nd Edition

INDEX

Criteria in home health nursing practice, [2007] (cont'd)
   implementation, 126
   leadership, 141–142
   outcomes identification, 123–124
   planning, 125
   prescriptive authority and treatment, 130
   professional practice evaluation, 135
   quality of practice, 132–133
   research, 139
   resource utilization, 140

Critical thinking in home health nursing practice, ix, 12, 91, 100. *See also* Evidence-based practice and research

D

Data and information in home health nursing practice, 8, 10, 19, 20, 22, 31, 34, 37, 38, 40, 46, 51, 53, 65. *See also* Electronic health records; Information technology
   collection, 22, 40, 44, 98, 121, 139

Decision-making in home health nursing practice, 6

Delegation in home health nursing practice, 15, 28–29, 73

Diagnosis in home health nursing practice, 8, 14
   competencies involving, 45, 46, 49, 58
   Standard of Practice, 46
      [2007], 122

Diagnosis-related groups (DRGs), 2

Disease management *see* Self-management

Dock, Lavinia, 1

Documentation, 13, 15, 19, 38
   competencies involving, 45, 46, 47, 50, 52, 53, 58, 65, 71
   electronic, 22, 28, 37

DRGs. *See* Diagnosis-related groups (DRGs)

E

Economic controls. *See* Cost and economic controls

Education in home health nursing practice, 6
   competencies involving, 62–63
   healthcare consumers, 16, 21, 26, 36, 55, 67, 104, 116, 128
   Standard of Professional Performance, 62–63
      [2007], 134. *See also* Educational preparation; Health teaching and health promotion

Educational preparation of home health nurses, 10–11
   of different nursing levels, 11–14

EHR. *See* Electronic health records (EHRs)

Electronic health records (EHRs) in home health nursing practice, 22, 24, 34, 35, 37–38, 45, 77

End of life issues in home health nursing practice, 5, 9, 28
   See also Hospice and palliative care

Environment in home health nursing practice. *See* Practice environments and settings; Environmental health

Environmental assessment in home health nursing practice, 8. *See also* Assessment

Environmental health in home health nursing practice
   competencies involving, 75–76
   Standard of Professional Performance, 75–76

Ethics in home health nursing practice, 27–31
   competencies involving, 45, 47, 60–61, 65
   Standard of Professional Performance, 60–61
      [2007], 138

Evaluation in home health nursing
practice, 10, 15, 19, 20
competencies involving, 58–59
Standard of Practice, 55, 57, 58–59,
65, 66, 73
[2007], 131
See also Professional practice
evaluation

Evidence-based practice and research
in home health nursing practice,
9, 12, 14, 18, 20, 21, 23, 26,
40, 139
competencies involving, 30,
33, 47, 48, 50, 51, 53, 64
defined, 77
Standard of Professional
Performance, 64
See also Research

Evolution of home health nursing
practice, 1–4, 93–94

Expected outcomes in home health
nursing practice, 9, 10, 46, 47–48,
49, 58
See also Outcomes identification

F

Families in home health nursing
practice, 3, 4, 5, 6, 7, 9, 14, 16, 17, 25,
27, 28, 33, 39, 44. *See also* Healthcare
consumers
defined, 77

Financial issues in home health nursing
practice, 7, 15, 23, 25, 26, 27
competencies involving, 44, 49, 61
finance and reimbursement issues,
39–40
resource utilization and, 73–74
See also Cost and economic controls

Frequency and duration, home health
nursing, 6

Functional assessments in home
health nursing practice, 8. *See also*
Assessment

Future of Nursing report, 13

G

Graduate-level prepared home health
nurse, 13
assessment competencies, 45
collaboration competencies, 70–71
consultation competencies, 56
coordination of care competencies, 53
diagnosis competencies, 46
education competencies, 63
environmental health competencies,
75–76
ethics competencies, 61
evaluation competencies, 58–59
evidence-based practice and research
competencies, 64
health teaching and health promotion
competencies, 54–55
implementation competencies, 52
leadership competencies, 69
outcomes identification
competencies, 47–48
planning competencies, 50
prescriptive authority and treatment
competencies, 57
professional practice evaluation
competencies, 72
quality of practice competencies, 66
resource utilization competencies, 74

*A Guide to District Nurses and Home
Visiting*, 1

H

Health coaches and coaching in home
health nursing practice, 7, 9, 26, 28,
32, 67
nurse coaches and coaching defined, 78

Health information records and
technology, 22, 55
See also Electronic health records
(EHR); Informatics; Information
technology

Health Information Technology for
Economic and Clinical Health
(HITECH), 37

INDEX

Health teaching and health promotion in home health nursing practice, 6–7
  competencies involving, 54–55
  nurse coaching and teaching, 9, 16, 28
  Standard of Practice, 54–55
    [2007], 128. *See also* Health coaches and coaching

Healthcare consumers, 5, 6, 7–8, 69, 136. *See also* Families
  education, 16, 21, 26, 36, 55, 67, 104, 116, 128

HHNA. *See* Home Healthcare Nurses Association (HHNA)

HITECH. *See* Health Information Technology for Economic and Clinical Health (HITECH)

Home care, 5

Home health agencies. *See* Agencies in home health nusing practice

Home health nurses, 5, 11–12
  as administrator, 18–19
  advanced practice (*See* Advanced practice registered nurses (APRNs))
  clinical educator, 20–22
  educational preparation of, 10–11, 99
  informatics liaison nurse, 22
  minimum qualifications, 12, 100
  quality and performance improvement nurse, 20
  as supervisor/clinical manager, 19–20

Home Health Nursing: Scope and Standards of Practice, Second Edition, ix, x

Home health nursing practice
  certification in, 11
  defined, 5
  distinguishing characteristics, 6–7
  educational preparation, 10–11
  ethics, 27–31
  evolution of, 1–4, 93–94
  finances and reimbursement, 39–40
  frequency and duration, 6
  goal of, 4, 5, 6
  informatics in, 35–39
  information technology and telehealth, 23, 35, 37–38, 40
  legal obligations and licensure, 111–112
  nursing shortage, 112
  patient population in, 3
  practice environments, 23–27
  process, 7–10, 96–99
  regulations, 111
  research, 31–35, 117–120
  roles and responsibilities, 11–22
  scope of practice, 4
    [2007], 87–154
  standardized terminologies and outcomes management, 38, 112–114
  trends, issues, and opportunities, 23–40, 107

Home Healthcare Nurse, x

Home Healthcare Nurses Association (HHNA), x, 10

Hospice care in home health nursing practice. *See* Palliative and hospice care

Hospitalization issues. *See* Rehospitalization issues

I

IADLs. *See* Independent activities of daily living (IADLs)

Implementation in home health nursing practice, 9–10
  competencies involving, 51–52
  Standard of Practice, 51–52
    [2007], 126

In-home message devices in home health nursing practice, 36

Independent activities of daily living (IADLs), 8

Informatics in home health nursing practice, 35–39

Informatics liaison nurse, 22

Information technology in home health nursing practice, 22, 23, 35, 37–38, 40, 54. *See also* Data and information; Electronic health records (EHRs); Informatics

Interdisciplinary practice in home health nursing, 31, 97, 100, 103, 117, 133, 136

Interprofessional practice in home health nursing, 5, 6, 8, 9, 12, 14, 16, 23, 49
defined, 77

Issues in home health nursing practice. *See* Trends, issues, and opportunities

J

Judgment in home health nursing practice, 13, 29, 62, 63, 69. *See also* Knowledge, skills, abilities, and judgment

K

Knowledge, skills, abilities, and judgment in home health nursing practice, 6. *See also* Critical thinking; Education; Evidence-based practice and research
assessment and, 44, 45
collaboration and, 70
education and, 62, 63
environmental health, 75
evidence-based practice and research, 64
implementation and, 51, 52
leadership and, 69
planning and, 50
prescriptive authority and treatment, 57

L

Laws and regulations in home health nursing practice, 19, 20, 31, 34, 35, 40, 57, 60, 73

Leadership in home health nursing practice
administrator roles and, 18–22
competencies involving, 68–69
informatics liaison nurse roles and, 22
Standard of Professional Performance, 68–69
[2007], 141–142

Legal issues in home health nursing practice. *See* Laws and regulations

Licensed practical nurse/licensed vocational nurse (LPN/LVN), 10, 15

LPN/LVN. *See* Licensed practical nurse/licensed vocational nurse

M

Magnet Recognition Program, 24

Meaningful use, 37
defined, 78

Measurement criteria. *See* Criteria

Medical home, defined, 78

Medicare, 2

Medication assessments in home health nursing practice, 8. *See also* Assessment

Metropolitan Life Insurance Company, 2

Minimum qualifications, home health nurses, 12, 100

N

NAHC. *See* National Association for Home Care and Hospice (NAHC)

NANDA. *See* North American Nursing Diagnosis Association (NANDA) International

National Association for Home Care and Hospice (NAHC), x, 3

National League for Nursing (NLN), 2

NIC. *See* Nursing Interventions Classification (NIC)

Nightingale, Florence, 1

INDEX

NLN. *See* National League for Nursing (NLN)

NOC. *See* Nursing Outcomes Classification (NOC)

North American Nursing Diagnosis Association (NANDA) International, 38

Notes on Nursing, 1

NPs. *See* Nurse practitioners (NPs)

Nurse coach, defined, 78. *See also* Health coaches and coaching

Nurse coaching, defined, 78. *See also* Health coaches and coaching

Nurse practitioners (NPs), 14, 102

Nursing: Scope and Standards of Practice, Second Edition, ix, 11

Nursing education. *See* Education

Nursing Interventions Classification (NIC), 38

Nursing Outcomes Classification (NOC), 38

Nursing process in home health nursing practice, 7–10, 12, 15, 17, 51, 65. *See also* Standards of Practice

Nursing's Social Policy Statement: The Essence of the Profession, ix, 91

O

OASIS. *See* Outcome and Assessment Information Set (OASIS)

Omaha System in home health nursing practice, 34–35, 118

Opportunities in home health nursing practice. *See* Trends, issues, and opportunities

Organizations/agencies in home health nursing practice, 2–3, 23, 24

Outcome and Assessment Information Set (OASIS), 34, 119

Outcomes,

Outcomes identification in home health nursing practice, 8–9, 97
 competencies involving, 47–48
 expected outcomes and, 46, 47–48
 Standard of Practice, 47–48
  [2007], 123–124
  See also Expected outcomes

Outcomes management in home health nursing practice, 33, 34, 38, 112–114

P

Palliative and hospice care in home health nursing practice, 3, 11, 13, 49
 review of studies of, 33
 end-of-life issues, 5, 9, 28

Pathway to Excellence Program, 24

Patient advocacy in home health nursing practice, 17

Patient-centered care in home health nursing practice, 26

Patient education in home health nursing practice, 6, 16

Patient engagement in home health nursing practice, 39–40
 defined, 78

Patient population in home health nursing practice, 3

Patient Protection and Affordable Care Act. *See* Affordable Care Act

Patient self-care; Patient self management. *See* Self-care; Self management.

Peer review and relations in home health nursing practice, 29, 72

Personal computers in home health nursing practice, 36

Personal health records (PHRs), 37. *See also* Electronic health records (EHRs)

Phone technology in home health nursing practice, 36

Physical assessment in home health nursing practice, 7. *See also* Assessment

Plan of care (POC), 15
  ethics and, 27, 28, 30
  See also Planning
Planning in home health nursing practice, 9, 97–98
  competencies involving, 49–50, 51, 52, 53, 59, 70, 73
  Standard of Practice, 49–50
  [2007], 125
POC. *See* Plan of care (POC)
Policies in home health nursing practice, 19, 22, 31, 32, 93, 98, 103
PPS. *See* Prospective payment system (PPS)
Practice environments and settings for home health nursing practice, 23–27, 29. *See also* Health teaching and health promotion
  safe work environments, 23, 24–25, 54
Prescriptive authority and treatment in home health nursing practice
  competencies involving, 57
  Standard of Practice, 57
  [2007], 130
Privacy in home health nursing practice. *See* Confidentiality and privacy
Professional practice evaluation in home health nursing practice
  competencies involving, 72
  Standard of Professional Performance, 72
  [2007], 135
Prospective payment system (PPS), 3
Psychosocial assessment in home health nursing practice, 7. *See also* Assessment

Q

Qualifications required, home health nurses, 12
Quality of care and patient outcomes, 14, 19, 21, 23, 24, 29, 33, 36, 37, 68
Quality improvement, 7, 14, 22, 23, 35, 38
Quality and performance improvement nurse, 20
Quality of life, 4, 5, 53
Quality of practice in home health nursing practice
  competencies involving, 65–66
  Standard of Professional Performance, 65–66
  [2007], 132–133

R

Rathbone, William, 1
Recipient of care. *See* Healthcare consumers
Regional health information organization (RHIO), 117
Registered nurses (RNs) in home health nursing practice, x, 92
  competencies, 44–45, 46, 47, 49–50, 51–52, 53, 54, 58, 60–61, 62, 64, 65–66, 67, 68–69, 70, 72, 73, 75
Regulatory requirements in home health nursing practice. *See also* Laws and regulations
Rehospitalization issues in home health nursing practice, 28, 32, 36, 40
  hospitalization rates and, 31–32, 34, 36
Reimbursement in home health nursing practice, 3, 7, 39–40
Research in home health nursing practice, 31–35
  research programs, 33–35
  Standard of Professional Performance [2007], 139
Resource utilization in home health nursing practice
  competencies involving, 73–74
  Standard of Professional Performance, 73–74
  [2007], 140

INDEX

Respect in home health nursing practice, 27

Responsibilities in home health nursing practice, 11–22, 28–29

RHIO. *See* Regional health information organization (RHIO)

Risks and risk management in home health nursing practice. *See also* Safety
competencies involving, 45, 46, 47, 54, 55, 56, 61, 67, 73, 75
nurse risks, 25
patient risks, 8, 31–32, 34

RNs. *See* Registered nurses (RNs)

Roles and responsibilities in home health nursing practice, 7, 11–22
administrative roles, 18–22
APRNs, 13
clinical roles, 15–17
CNSs, 13–14
graduate-level prepared home health nurse, 13
home health nurse, 11–12
NPs, 14

S

Safety in home health nursing practice, 8, 12, 17, 22, 32, 33, 35. *See also* Risks and risk management
competencies involving, 46, 51, 52, 53, 60, 65, 71
environmental health and, 75
ethics and, 27, 28, 29, 30
safe work environments, 23, 24–25, 54

Sanger, Margaret, 1

Scope and Standards of Home Health Nursing Practice, ix

Scope of home health nursing practice, 4
[2007], 87–154

Self-care management, 5, 9, 16, 32, 44, 54, 70

Self-management, of disease by patients, 6, 12, 51, 63

Settings for home health nursing practice. *See* Practice environments and settings

Shortage, nursing, 112

Skills in home health nursing practice. *See* Knowledge, skills, abilities, and judgment

Social Security Amendments, 2

Standardized terminologies in home health nursing practice, 38, 112–114

Standards. *See also* Standards of Practice; Standards of Professional Performance
significance of, 43

Standards of Home Health Nursing Practice, ix, 3, 91

Standards of Practice for Home Health Nursing. *See also* Standards of Professional Performance for Home Health Nursing; Specific standard
assessment, 44–45
consultation, 56
coordination of care, 53
diagnosis, 46
evaluation, 58–59
health teaching and health promotion, 54–55
implementation, 51–52
outcomes identification, 47–48
planning, 49–50
prescriptive authority and treatment, 57
[2007], 121–131

Standards of Professional Performance for Home Health Nursing. *See also* Standards of Practice for Home Health Nursing; Specific standard
collaboration, 70–71
communication, 67
education, 62–63
environmental health, 75–76
ethics, 60–61
evidence-based practice and research, 64
leadership, 68–69

INDEX

professional practice evaluation, 72
quality of practice, 65–66
resource utilization, 73–74
[2007], 132–142

Supervisor/clinical manager in home health nursing practice, 19–20

T

Teaching in home health nursing practice. *See* Health teaching and health promotion

Teams and teamwork, 2, 9, 12, 16, 22, 29, 31, 49, 64, 65, 67, 70. *See also* Interdisciplinary practice; Interprofessional practice

Technological improvements in home health nursing practice, 23, 35, 36, 40 *See also* Information technology

Telehealth in home health nursing practice, 35–36

Telemonitors in home health nursing practice, 36

Terminologies in home health nursing practice, 38, 112–114

Transitional care in home health nursing practice, 34

Treatment in home health nursing practice. *See* Prescriptive authority and treatment

Trends, issues, and opportunities in home health nursing practice, 3–4, 23–40
ethics, 27–31
finances and reimbursement, 39–40
informatics, 35–39
practice environments, 23–27
research, 31–35

V

Values, attitudes, and beliefs in home health nursing practice, 16, 18, 27, 29, 31, 44, 55, 60

Video cameras in home health nursing practice, 36, 116

Video conferencing in home health nursing practice, 36, 116

Visiting Nurse Associations (VNAs), 1, 118–119

Visiting Nurse Associations of America (VNAA), 3

VNAA. *See* Visiting Nurse Associations of America (VNAA)

VNAs. *See* Visiting Nurse Associations (VNAs)

W

Wald, Lillian, 1

Work and practice environments for home health nursing practice. *See* Practice environments and settings